st Facts

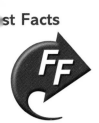

Fast Fac
Ophthalmology

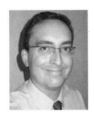

Anthony Pane MBBS(Hons) MMedSc FRANZCO
Consultant Ophthalmic Surgeon
Mater Hospital
Brisbane, Australia

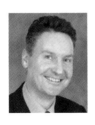

Peter Simcock MBChB MRCP FRCS FRCOphth DO
Consultant Ophthalmic Surgeon
West of England Eye Unit
Exeter, Devon, UK

Declaration of Independence

This book is as balanced and as practical as we can make it.

Ideas for improvement are always welcome:

feedback@fastfacts.com

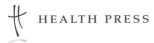
HEALTH PRESS

Fast Facts: Ophthalmology
First published May 2006

Text © 2006 Anthony Pane, Peter Simcock
© 2006 in this edition Health Press Limited
Health Press Limited, Elizabeth House, Queen Street, Abingdon,
Oxford OX14 3LN, UK
Tel: +44 (0)1235 523233
Fax: +44 (0)1235 523238

Book orders can be placed by telephone or via the website.
For regional distributors or to order via the website, please go to:
www.fastfacts.com
For telephone orders, please call 01752 202301 (UK), +44 1752 202301 (Europe),
1 800 247 6553 (USA, toll free) or +1 419 281 1802 (Canada).

Fast Facts is a trademark of Health Press Limited.

The publisher and the authors have made every effort to ensure the accuracy of this
book, but cannot accept responsibility for any errors or omissions.

For all drugs, please consult the product labeling approved in your country for
prescribing information.

A CIP record for this title is available from the British Library.

ISBN 1-903734-64-9 (978-1-903734-64-3)

Pane (Anthony)
Fast Facts: Ophthalmology/
Anthony Pane, Peter Simcock

Medical illustrations by Dee McLean, London, UK.
Typesetting and page layout by Zed, Oxford, UK.
Printed by LinneyPrint, Mansfield, UK.

Printed with vegetable inks on fully biodegradable and
recyclable paper manufactured from sustainable forests.

Low
chlorine

Sustainable
forests

NORDIC ENVIRONMENTAL LABEL
444   001
Low emissions
during production

Glossary

Amaurosis fugax: transient, painless loss of vision in one eye with complete recovery of vision, usually within minutes; most commonly caused by embolism from a stenosed carotid artery

Amblyopia: reduced vision in an eye that has not functioned well during early childhood; most often occurs as a result of eye misalignment or focusing error that is not identified and treated early in childhood

Anisocoria: unequal pupil size

ARMD: age-related macular degeneration – a degenerative condition of the macula (central retina), which results in a deterioration of central vision

Blepharitis: inflammation of the eyelids

Chalazion: a slow-growing lump on the eyelid caused by inflammation of oil glands

Ectropion: the lower eyelid is turned out and hangs away from the eyeball

Entropion: the lower eyelid is turned in, with the eyelashes rubbing on the eyeball

Epiphora: watering of one or both eyes, without eye pain, irritation or redness

Exophthalmos: another term for proptosis (see below)

Foreign body sensation: the patient says 'It feels like something is in my eye'; causes include corneal or conjunctival foreign body, foreign body under the upper lid, inturned eyelashes, corneal ulcer or corneal abrasion

Hemianopia: loss of vision in one half of the visual field of one or both eyes, across to the vertical midline; this often signifies disease of the brain's visual pathways

Hyphema: collection of blood in the anterior chamber of the eye (between the iris and cornea)

Hypopyon: collection of pus in the anterior chamber of the eye

Iritis: autoimmune inflammation in the anterior chamber of the eye

Metamorphopsia: the visual symptom of distortion of straight lines or shapes

Papilledema: swelling of both optic nerve heads caused by increased intracranial pressure (e.g. due to a brain tumor)

Proptosis: forward displacement of the eye (causing a 'bulging' appearance)

Ptosis: drooping upper eyelid

RAPD: relative afferent pupillary defect – an abnormal response to the swinging light test, signifying serious retinal or optic nerve disease

Scotoma: absent or diminished vision in an isolated area of the visual field

Slit-lamp microscope: table-mounted microscope with attached light that enables examination of the surface and interior of a patient's eye at high magnification

Thyroid eye disease: orbital disease associated with idiopathic hyperthyroidism (Graves' disease), which can cause red eyes, lid retraction, proptosis, or double or blurred vision

TIA: Transient ischemic attack – a brief episode of neurological disturbance caused by a reduced supply of blood to an area of the brain

VA: visual acuity – clarity of central vision, measured on a vision chart, one eye at a time

Visual field: the total area visible with one eye, without moving the eye

Introduction

As a primary care provider you will not find it possible to diagnose the majority of eye diseases accurately. This is because the eye is so small and so complex that only careful examination with a slit-lamp microscope and a retinal lens can provide a true diagnosis of most patients' eye complaints.

So what can you do? Patients see you almost every day with eye problems and expect you to be able to help them. This book will help you triage your eye patients into three groups:

- those with serious eye emergencies, who require urgent referral to an ophthalmologist (to be seen the same day)
- those who do not have urgent problems, but require routine referral
- those you can either observe or treat yourself.

Fortunately, a brief history and examination (even with just a visual acuity chart and a flashlight) can almost always differentiate between these three groups. However, you have to know what to ask and what to look for to determine the urgency of each case.

This book is organized by patient presentation (e.g. red eye, blurred vision, double vision) rather than by disease, to facilitate rapid reference in clinical practice. Each chapter describes the essential management steps for each presenting symptom, in terms of referral or treatment options, followed by an overview of the common eye diseases that can cause such symptoms. Important issues are summarized in the key points at the end of each chapter.

Ophthalmology is one of the most difficult areas of primary care and is full of pitfalls for even the most diligent of doctors. We hope this book helps you avoid the traps.

Acknowledgments. Anthony Pane gratefully acknowledges financial assistance from the Prevent Blindness Foundation through Viertels Vision in the preparation of this book, and would like to thank Des, Jan, Sara and Kath for their ongoing encouragement and support. Peter Simcock thanks Moira and Leona for their unremitting support and dedicates this book to the memory of Les and Ken.

1   Eye examination

You only have a few minutes with each patient who comes to see you with an eye complaint, and (if you're a general practitioner) you probably have very little eye examination equipment. A careful history of the patient's eye symptoms plus looking for a few critical signs of serious disease will help you identify how urgently the patient should be referred to an ophthalmologist, or whether you can treat them yourself.

Eye anatomy

The eye, its surrounding structures and the brain's visual pathways can be affected by a wide spectrum of clinical conditions. Fortunately, the cornea and the ocular media are transparent, so most of the eyeball itself can be observed directly for signs of abnormality. Figure 1.1 depicts the essential components of the eye's optical system, many of which are referred to throughout the rest of this book. The main stages of an eye assessment are listed in Table 1.1 and are discussed in more detail below.

Taking a history

When a patient presents with an eye complaint, you will need to find out the exact nature and severity of the problem. Questions to ask include:

- Do you have blurred vision, and if so, is it in one or both eyes?
- Which part of the vision is affected?
- How sudden was the onset?
- What has happened since – has it improved, worsened or stayed the same?
- Do you have any other eye symptoms, for example, pain, sensitivity to light, flashes or floaters?

You will then need to ask about:

- the patient's ophthalmic history
- the patient's medical and surgical history
- the medications they are currently taking
- any family history of eye problems.

(a)

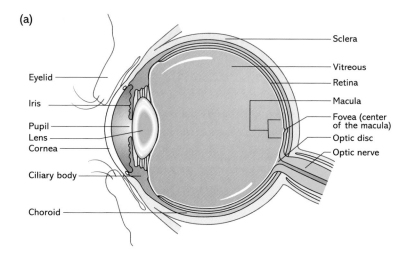

- Sclera
- Vitreous
- Retina
- Macula
- Fovea (center of the macula)
- Optic disc
- Optic nerve
- Eyelid
- Iris
- Pupil
- Lens
- Cornea
- Ciliary body
- Choroid

(b)

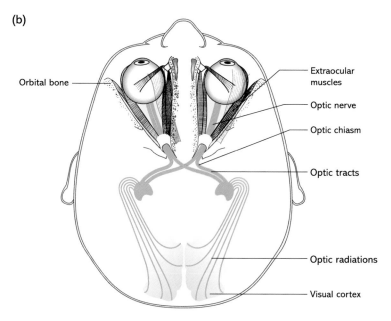

- Orbital bone
- Extraocular muscles
- Optic nerve
- Optic chiasm
- Optic tracts
- Optic radiations
- Visual cortex

Figure 1.1 Basic eye anatomy. (a) Main eye structures. (b) View from above, showing the visual pathway. Information leaves the eye via nerve fibers that form the optic nerve. The fibers partially cross at the optic chiasm, then continue as the optic tracts, before fanning out as optic radiations to reach the visual cortex at the back of the brain.

Presenting complaint. Spending a minute to clarify the exact nature of the patient's eye complaint and its development over time often gives the best clues to a likely diagnosis.

Are the symptoms in one or both eyes? If blurred vision or field loss is definitely localized to one eye, the disease is in that eye (or its optic nerve); however, if symptoms are bilateral, disease could be present in both eyes, or in the optic chiasm or retrochiasmal pathway in the brain. Patients with homonymous hemianopic field loss may attribute the problem only to the eye with the temporal (ear-side) field loss; for example, a patient with a left occipital stroke may erroneously complain of field loss in the right eye only.

What is the exact nature of the symptom? Is it blurred vision, visual field loss (a blank or blurry patch in the central or peripheral vision), pain, redness, irritation, foreign body sensation ('something is in my eye') or double vision?

Blurred vision or field loss. Ask the patient about each eye: 'Where is the vision blurry: all over, just in the center or mainly out to one side?'

TABLE 1.1

Principal elements of the basic eye assessment

History	Examination
Presenting complaint	Visual acuity (VA)
Ophthalmic history	Visual fields
Medical and surgical history	Eye movements
	Pupil size and reaction (including swinging light test)
Medications	
Family history	Eyelids
	Eye surface
	Optic discs and retina (by ophthalmoscopy)
	Intraocular pressure (by tonometer, if available)
	Higher magnification examination (by slit-lamp microscope, if available)

Asking the patient to cover one eye at a time and to report what they see while they look at your nose can be very useful. If only the patch around your nose is blurry and the rest is clear, the patient probably has a central scotoma from macular or optic nerve disease; if half of your face is clear and the other half is blurry, they may have a chiasmal or retrochiasmal stroke or tumor. New-onset flashes and/or floating spots in one eye usually indicate posterior vitreous detachment, vitreous hemorrhage or retinal tear which may result in retinal detachment. Distortion at the center of vision (metamorphopsia) is most commonly due to age-related macular degeneration.

Pain. A 'scratchy' pain at the front of the eye often indicates a corneal or subtarsal foreign body or corneal ulcer, whereas a deep ache inside the eye may suggest iritis or acute glaucoma.

Eye injury. It is important to get a clear idea of the mechanism of injury. If something hit the eye, find out what it was and with what velocity it struck the eye. Patients who give a history of being struck in the eye with a fragment of high-speed metal, or those who have received sharp trauma to the eye, need urgent referral for a slit-lamp examination and an X-ray to determine whether a perforating injury, with or without an intraocular foreign body, is present, even if the results of your examination are normal.

Red eye. It is important to ask specific questions to find out whether the patient has a 'good' or 'bad' red eye (see Chapter 2 – red eye): does the patient have blurred vision, pain or photophobia? If the patient has any of these symptoms, and you can't find a corneal foreign body or other easily treatable explanation for the red eye, it is a 'bad' red eye and needs urgent ophthalmic referral.

Tracking symptom development. For all eye complaints, after the symptoms have been accurately identified it is important to track the development of each symptom over time.

- When did it start?
- How rapidly did it start? The speed of onset can sometimes be a guide to the nature of the disease; for example, very sudden visual loss over seconds or minutes is often due to a vascular occlusion.
- What has happened since: is it getting better or worse, or staying the same?

Practitioners should also remain aware of symptoms associated with temporal arteritis, a potentially bilaterally blinding disease that only occurs in patients over the age of 50 (see page 54).

Ophthalmic history. A patient who has recently had eye surgery and presents with a red eye or blurred vision obviously needs urgent referral. Patients with a more remote history of eye disease or surgery are also more likely to develop problems in the future. All patients with a red eye should be asked if they wear contact lenses, as this greatly increases the risk of an infective corneal ulcer.

Medical and surgical history

Diabetes. A diabetic patient complaining of the acute or subacute onset of blurred vision, floaters or field loss should always be taken seriously and referred urgently; patients with diabetes have a high risk of serious eye disease, including diabetic maculopathy, vitreous hemorrhage and traction retinal detachment. It is essential that every diabetic in your practice has regular screening for diabetic retinopathy, even if they are visually asymptomatic.

Cardiovascular complaints. Patients with hypertension or carotid stenosis may develop a retinal vascular occlusion.

Graves' disease. Patients with Graves' disease can develop proptosis and double vision from swelling of the extraocular muscles. They are also at risk of compressive optic neuropathy from pressure on the optic nerve that causes blurring of vision.

Medications. Does the patient take any eye drops or tablets for their eyes? If so, what are they for? You should also check whether the patient is taking any medications that can cause eye damage, e.g. antituberculosis antibiotics (ethambutol and isoniazid), tamoxifen or vigabatrin.

Family history. If first-degree relatives have suffered from glaucoma, retinal detachment or other serious eye diseases, the patient is often at greater risk of developing these conditions. Any patient who has a close relative with glaucoma should, from early adulthood, commence regular glaucoma screening examinations performed by an optometrist.

Examination

When performing a basic eye examination you will need to assess:

- visual acuity (VA)
- visual field
- eye movements (if the patient has a 'turned eye' or double vision)
- pupil size and reaction (including the swinging light test; see page 16)
- eyelids
- eye surface
- optic discs and retina (by ophthalmoscopy)
- intraocular pressure (by tonometer, if available)
- individual components of the eye at higher magnification (by slit-lamp microscope, if available).

Visual acuity (VA). Every general practice should have a distance VA chart for testing the sharpness of vision at 6 m (20 ft) (Figure 1.2), and every patient complaining of blurred vision should ideally have their VA tested. VA is tested one eye at a time, with the patient wearing their 'distance' glasses. If acuity is poor, the patient should remove their glasses and read the chart through a 'pinhole'; you can use a commercial pinhole occluder or make one yourself by pushing the tip of a ballpoint pen through a sheet of paper. If VA improves through the pinhole, the patient may need a change of glasses, or a corneal scar or cataract could be present. If the patient cannot even see the largest letter on the chart, check whether they can:

- count your fingers from 1 m (3 ft) away – 'count fingers' vision
- see your hand moving – 'hand movements' vision
- see a bright light – if they can, 'perception of light'; if not, 'no perception of light'.

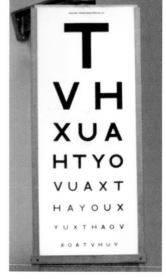

Figure 1.2 The distance visual acuity chart for testing vision at 6 m (20 ft).

Special techniques may be required to test young children's VA, such as assessing visual behavior and target tracking.

Visual field to confrontation. There is a lot more to vision than just visual acuity. Testing the visual field (the entire sideways extent of vision for each eye) is also important, as this can lead to the detection of disease that would be missed if VA alone were tested. For example, a patient with a pituitary tumor can have a bitemporal hemianopia but still retain normal VA in each eye.

To test the patient's right visual field to confrontation, sit directly in front of the patient and close your right eye, then ask the patient to cover their left eye with their left hand and to stare into your left eye. Hold up one, two or five fingers midway between yourself and the patient (up and right, up and left, down and right, and down and left) so that you can see them yourself while still staring into the patient's eye (Figure 1.3). Ask the patient how many fingers you are holding up. Then repeat the procedure on the left eye. There are many other tests for visual field, such as gradually bringing in a target from the periphery and asking the patient to tell you when they see it; with this technique, a neurological field defect may be detected earlier with a red target than with a white one.

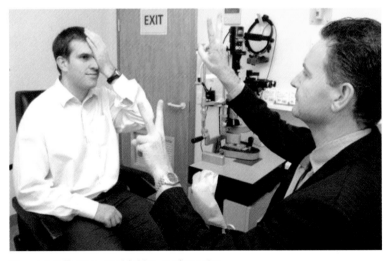

Figure 1.3 Testing visual field to confrontation.

Eye movements should be tested in patients who complain of double vision, or in children who present with a squint ('turned eye'). A detailed ocular motility assessment is much more complicated than simply asking the patient to 'follow my pen' and watching the extent of eye movement, although this will pick up large restrictions of movement.

We do not have room in this book for a full discussion of eye movement testing, but here is a brief overview of the main tests. First, assess eye alignment in the primary position (looking straight ahead) for both distant and near targets. A misalignment may be obvious or it may be detectable only during a cover test (in which one eye at a time is covered and uncovered while you look for movement of the other eye). The deviation while the patient is looking straight ahead may be:

- esotropia (one eye turned in)
- exotropia (one eye turned out)
- hypertropia (one eye turned up)
- hypotropia (one eye turned down)
- an oblique deviation.

Next, ask the patient to keep their head still and follow a slowly moving target with their eyes (right, up and right, up, up and left, left, down and left, down, down and right), while you look for any restriction in the normal range of movement of one or both eyes.

Pupils. It is important to note the pupil size in each eye and whether each pupil constricts briskly to a bright light in a dimly lit room. However, the most important test is the 'swinging light test', which is used to look for a relative afferent pupillary defect (RAPD) (Figure 1.4). This should be performed for all patients complaining of blurred vision, flashes, floaters or visual field loss. Dim the room lights and use a bright light source (such as a bright flashlight or an ophthalmoscope); ask the patient to stare at a distant target and swing the light repeatedly between the two eyes, shining it for 1–2 seconds in each eye. A normal response is for each pupil to constrict when the light is shone on each eye in turn. An RAPD (the abnormal response) occurs when one pupil dilates, rather than constricts, when the light is shone on it. If an RAPD is found, serious retinal or optic nerve disease on the same side is likely.

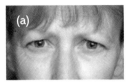
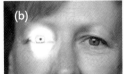
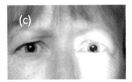

Figure 1.4 Testing for a relative afferent pupillary defect (RAPD) using the swinging light test: (a) normal size of pupils with room lights on; (b) room lights are turned down, the patient looks into the distance and a light is shone onto the right eye – the patient shows a normal response, with constriction of both pupils; (c) dilation of both pupils after suddenly swinging the light to the left eye, indicating a left RAPD.

Eyelid and eye surface examination

White light. Examine the eyes and eyelids with a flashlight and, if you have one, a magnifier (Figure 1.5a). You will need to take note of a number of features.

- Are the eyes red?
- Are the corneas clear?
- Is there a corneal or conjunctival foreign body?
- Are the pupils regular in shape and equal in size?

Blue light and fluorescein drops. For cases of red eye, it is useful to administer the orange dye fluorescein (unless you think the patient has a penetrating injury, in which case no drops should be used). Instill a drop of fluorescein in the eye, or put a drop of saline on a fluorescein paper strip and touch it to the lower conjunctiva. Then examine the corneal and conjunctival surface with a bright blue light in a dark room (Figure 1.5b). If you don't have a commercial blue filter for your flashlight, blue cellophane held over the flashlight can be used instead.

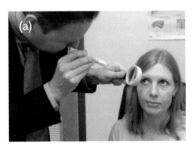
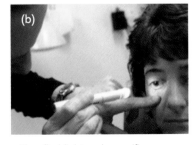

Figure 1.5 (a) Examining the eye surface with a flashlight and magnifier; (b) examining with a blue light and fluorescein drops.

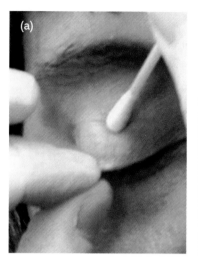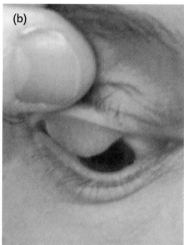

Figure 1.6 (a) Everting the upper eyelid by gently pulling it away from the eye and pushing down with a cotton swab (cotton bud); (b) checking the underside of the upper lid when fully everted.

A corneal ulcer or abrasion will show up as a fluorescent yellow-green area on the cornea (see page 93). Ulcers that are invisible under white light can be detected by this procedure.

Eyelid examination. Examine the eyelids carefully and check that they are in the normal position, that is, not turned in or out. If the patient complains of a foreign body sensation ('something is in my eye'), but you can't see a corneal ulcer or foreign body, it is important to evert ('flip') the eyelid to see if anything is trapped between the upper or lower eyelid and the eyeball. Pull the lower eyelid downwards and look behind it with a flashlight. To evert the upper eyelid, pull it away from the eye, holding onto the lashes, and push down onto the upper skin surface with a cotton swab (cotton bud) (Figure 1.6a) until the lid flips over (Figure 1.6b).

Intraocular pressure testing. There are various methods of testing intraocular pressure; instruments that measure eye pressure are called tonometers. All patients with a red eye and blurred vision, pain or photophobia need urgent pressure testing by an ophthalmologist to exclude acute glaucoma.

Ophthalmoscopy becomes easier and more accurate if you use dilating eye drops, such as tropicamide 1%, before examination. However, you should only administer these drops to adults, and must warn them that their vision will be blurred and that they should not drive for 8 hours. The drops should not be used in patients with acute neurological problems.

Intraocular examination with the direct ophthalmoscope is best taught in practice. The procedure follows two key stages.

- Check the red reflex.
- Examine the optic discs, retinal blood vessels and macula.

Red reflex. Set the lens wheel on '0', stand 1 m (3 ft) away from the patient in a dark room, look through the ophthalmoscope at the patient's eyes and ask them to look at the ophthalmoscope light. A normal red reflex (the reflection from inside the eye) is a uniform orange or red glow. Remember to examine the red reflex as part of all routine 'well baby' first neonatal checks to exclude congenital cataract or retinoblastoma.

Optic discs, retinal blood vessels and macula. Move close to the patient and view the optic disc in each eye, noting whether the disc looks normal or abnormal (Figure 1.7); trace the retinal blood vessels away from the disc. View as much of the peripheral retina as possible by asking the patient to look up, down, right and left in turn. Finally, ask the patient to look directly at the light to view the macula.

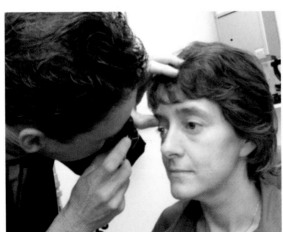

Figure 1.7
Examination of the optic disc and retina using the direct ophthalmoscope.

It is important to remember to examine the optic discs by direct ophthalmoscopy in all patients complaining of headache to see if bilateral disc swelling caused by raised intracranial pressure (papilledema) is present. Remember that although the direct ophthalmoscope gives good images of the optic discs it has only a very small field of view; a 'normal' direct ophthalmoscope examination therefore does not exclude the possibility of serious intraocular disease.

Slit-lamp examination is required to determine whether an eye is definitely 'normal'. A slit-lamp microscope provides a highly magnified three-dimensional view of the eye surface, anterior chamber, lens and, with handheld fundus lenses, the vitreous, retina and optic disc (Figure 1.8). There are many eye diseases, for example iritis, which can only be diagnosed with the slit lamp. Again, examination with this instrument is best taught in practice.

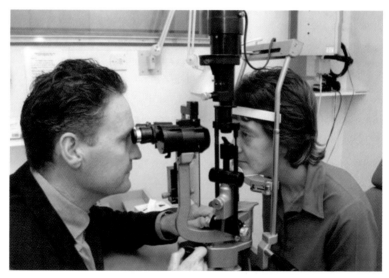

Figure 1.8 Eye examination by slit-lamp microscope.

Key points – eye examination

- Eye disease cannot be accurately diagnosed without a slit-lamp microscope examination.
- Carry out a basic eye assessment by:
  - identifying the presenting symptoms
  - taking a complete patient history
  - performing as thorough an examination as you can with the equipment you have available.
- Test visual acuity (VA) in every patient who complains of blurred vision.
- Test the visual field to confrontation to detect disease that would be missed by testing for VA alone.
- Perform the 'swinging light test' to check for a relative afferent pupillary defect (RAPD) in all patients who complain of blurred vision, flashes, floaters or visual field loss. The presence of an RAPD signifies serious retinal or optic nerve disease.
- In patients with red eye/s, the use of a blue light and fluorescein drops may identify a corneal ulcer that is invisible with white light alone.
- The commonly available handheld direct ophthalmoscope is not a particularly good instrument for examining the optic discs and retina. Patients with 'normal fundoscopy' with the direct ophthalmoscope can still have serious disease detectable only by examination with the slit-lamp microscope and retinal lenses.
- Use your patients' eye symptoms and signs to triage them according to their need for referral to an ophthalmologist: those with serious eye emergencies who require urgent referral, those with non-urgent problems who require routine referral and those whom you can observe or treat yourself.

Red eye is one of the most common eye symptoms your patients will complain of. Many diseases can result in a red eye, ranging from harmless but irritating complaints such as conjunctivitis, which you can treat yourself, to severe sight-threatening diseases such as acute glaucoma, which can be permanently blinding if you don't immediately refer the patient for emergency treatment. You must be able to recognize the severity of a red eye (that is, distinguish between a 'good' and 'bad' red eye), as outlined below. For red eye due to trauma (including corneal foreign body), see Chapter 10 – eye trauma.

'Bad' red eye

'Bad' red eye is defined as one red eye (rarely bilateral) of unknown cause with one or more of the 'five Ps', as detailed in Table 2.1.

TABLE 2.1

The '5 Ps' for diagnosis of a 'bad' red eye

- **P**ain

- **P**hotophobia (sensitivity to light)

- **P**oor vision (the patient complains of blurred vision or testing reveals decreased acuity)

- **P**us in the cornea or anterior chamber (corneal ulcer or hypopyon)

- **P**upil abnormality (such as abnormal size or shape, or poor constriction to light)

Any patient with red eye/s and one or more of the 'five Ps' must be referred immediately and urgently to an ophthalmologist. Do not give the patient any treatment.

The underlying cause of a 'bad' red eye, such as acute glaucoma or iritis, can only be diagnosed by a careful slit-lamp examination and measurement of intraocular pressure.

> Remember: not every red eye is 'conjunctivitis'. Misdiagnosing a 'bad' red eye as conjunctivitis can result in permanent blindness and a very angry patient!

'Good' red eye

'Good' red eye is diagnosed when one or both eyes are red, but:
- there is no pain, photophobia or blurred vision
- both eyes are otherwise completely normal on examination.

You can assess these patients for treatment yourself, or refer non-urgently to an ophthalmologist. The underlying cause could be viral, allergic or bacterial conjunctivitis, dry eyes or blepharitis. However, you should refer any patient with 'good' red eye if the eye has not improved within 2 weeks, or if it turns into 'bad' red eye at any stage.

Prescribing eye drops

The only eye drops you should prescribe without an ophthalmologist's opinion are artificial tears for dry eye, antibiotics for bacterial conjunctivitis and mast-cell inhibitors for allergic conjunctivitis.

Antibiotic eye drops should only be prescribed for bacterial conjunctivitis, which presents as:
- two 'good' red eyes
- a pus-like discharge
- no pain or photophobia, and normal vision.

Antibiotics will never help one red eye, as the diagnosis is either something serious (a 'bad' red eye), which should lead to immediate patient referral, or viral conjunctivitis, which will resolve spontaneously and is not helped by antibiotics.

Never prescribe steroid eye drops – except under instruction from an ophthalmologist – as they can exacerbate infections, and can cause cataracts and glaucoma.

Diseases that present as 'bad' red eye

For the conditions described in this section, urgent treatment by an ophthalmologist can often save the patient's sight. If referral is delayed, even by a few days, permanent visual loss can occur.

> Do not prescribe any treatment for 'bad' red eye – all of these conditions require urgent ophthalmic referral (to be seen the same day).

Iritis (anterior uveitis) is inflammation in the anterior chamber of the eye that can only be diagnosed by slit-lamp examination. Patients are usually young or middle-aged adults who present with one or more of: blurred vision (although vision can be normal early on), red eye (also mild in early cases), eye pain and photophobia.

The pupil may look normal, be irregular or be distorted. On slit-lamp examination, white cells can be seen in the anterior chamber and clumps of white cells (keratic precipitates) may be seen on the inside of the cornea (Figure 2.1).

Acute glaucoma is a sudden rise in intraocular pressure: normal pressure is less than 21 mmHg, but in acute glaucoma it is usually above 40 mmHg. Symptoms include eye ache or pain (which can be severe, can cause nausea or vomiting, and can be mistaken for migraine) and blurred vision, sometimes with haloes around lights.

The cornea may appear normal or cloudy, while the pupil may be normal or mid-dilated and unreactive (Figure 2.2). This disease can only

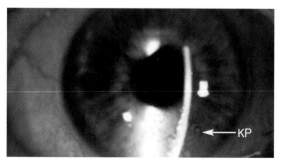

Figure 2.1 Iritis (inflammation in the anterior chamber of the eye). KP, keratic precipitates (small spots on the inside of the cornea).

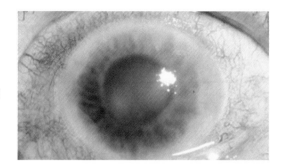

Figure 2.2 Acute glaucoma with hazy cornea and mid-dilated pupil.

be diagnosed by testing the eye's intraocular pressure with a tonometer. Acute glaucoma is more common in longsighted elderly patients.

Do not confuse this condition with the more common chronic glaucoma, in which there is no eye redness or pain, the patient is almost always asymptomatic and eye pressure is usually below 30 mmHg (see Chapter 3 – blurred vision).

Infective corneal ulcer. The cornea is normally completely clear, but in cases of infective corneal ulcer it is infiltrated by a virus, bacterium or fungus. This can occur in patients of all ages, particularly in individuals who wear contact lenses. There is usually eye pain or foreign body sensation; however, in herpetic dendritic ulcers the eye becomes numb (Figure 2.3), so even a large ulcer may not cause discomfort. Red eye, mildly or severely blurred vision, and photophobia are common.

A viral ulcer may be invisible unless fluorescein examination is performed, but bacterial or fungal ulcers usually cause a visible white infiltrate in the cornea (Figure 2.4). If severe, hypopyon (a fluid pus level in the inferior part of the anterior chamber) may be visible.

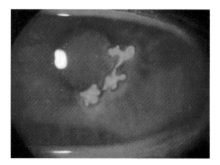

Figure 2.3 Dendritic ulcer due to herpes simplex virus infection, observed under blue light after administration of fluorescein dye drops.

Scleritis is inflammation of the normally white sclera (eye wall) (Figure 2.5). Patients complain of aching pain, which is often severe and can wake the patient at night. Vision can be normal or blurred. On examination, the sclera appears diffusely or focally red. The condition is often associated with rheumatoid arthritis or systemic vasculitis.

Endophthalmitis is a severe infection of the intraocular contents, which usually occurs within days or weeks of eye surgery. The infection causes blurred vision (sometimes with floaters), pain and photophobia, and there are signs of iritis and inflammation of the vitreous cavity (Figure 2.6).

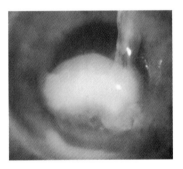

Figure 2.4 Infective corneal ulcer – the visible white infiltrate in the cornea indicates the presence of a bacterial or fungal infection; a small hypopyon is also present.

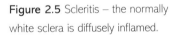

Figure 2.5 Scleritis – the normally white sclera is diffusely inflamed.

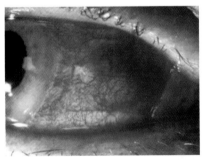

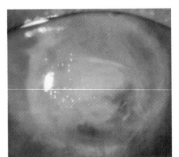

Figure 2.6 Endophthalmitis – severe infection of the intraocular contents.

Diseases that present as 'good' red eye

Obviously it is never *good* to have a red eye, but the conditions listed below are annoying rather than dangerous. However, 'bad' red-eye diseases sometimes present like this early on, so it is important to follow these patients and refer them immediately if their condition persists or deteriorates.

> Cases of 'good' red eye should be referred to an ophthalmologist if they do not start to improve within 2 weeks, or immediately if blurred vision, pain or photophobia develops.

Bacterial conjunctivitis almost always affects *both* eyes, although it can be briefly unilateral. The eyes are red, gritty and sticky, with a pus-like discharge (Figure 2.7). Lid eversion may show papillae (small, pink, cobblestone-like lumps). There is no need to take a microbiology swab. Treat with a topical antibiotic every 2 hours during the day for several days until improvement occurs, then four times a day for a week. Warn the patient that the condition is contagious.

Viral conjunctivitis is often caused by one of the common cold viruses, and patients often, but not always, have recently had a viral upper respiratory tract infection. One or both eyes become red, and

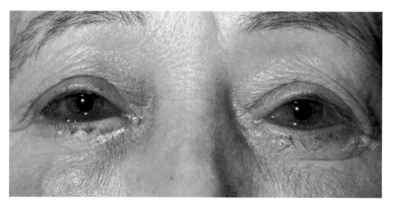

Figure 2.7 Bacterial conjunctivitis; the eyes are red, feel gritty and sticky and exude a pus-like discharge.

there is a clear watery discharge, without pus. Lid eversion can reveal
follicles, which look like small, gray grains of rice (Figure 2.8).
Pre-auricular or cervical lymphadenopathy may or may not be
present.

No treatment is of benefit and the infection will resolve with time.
Warn the patient that the infection is highly contagious until the
redness has subsided.

Allergic conjunctivitis most commonly occurs in patients with
asthma, eczema or hay fever, although it can occur in isolation. The
predominant symptom is itching of one or both eyes. There is either
no discharge, or a watery or scant, sticky discharge (Figure 2.9a); lid
eversion may show papillae (Figure 2.9b). The condition can be acute
and severe (often in association with a hay fever attack), seasonal (in
spring or summer) or chronic. Contact lens wearers can sometimes
have an allergy to one of their solutions.

If the patient wears contact lenses, they should see their contact lens
prescriber for a check-up. If not, prescribe mast-cell inhibitor drops
(e.g. cromoglycate, three times daily) to see whether they help. Warn
the patient that they may need to use the drops for several weeks
before they notice any improvement. Steroid eye drops will make the
eyes feel much better, but should only be prescribed on the advice of
an ophthalmologist, as long-term use can cause glaucoma and
cataracts.

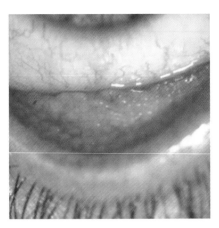

Figure 2.8 Viral conjunctivitis; the
eyes have a clear, watery
discharge but no pus; sometimes,
as shown in this picture, eversion
of the lower lid reveals follicles
(which look like small gray grains
of rice).

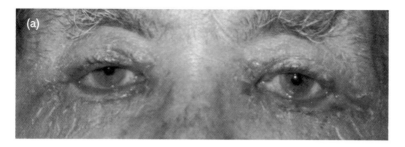

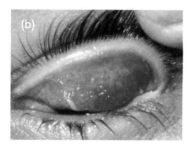

Figure 2.9 Allergic conjunctivitis: (a) red, itchy eyes with a scant, sticky discharge; (b) subtarsal papillae (small, pink cobblestone-like lumps seen on eyelid eversion).

Subconjunctival hemorrhage is usually spontaneous but can occur after a severe bout of coughing. Patients are often very alarmed by the condition, which presents as a large area of bright red blood between the conjunctiva and the underlying sclera (Figure 2.10). However, subconjunctival hemorrhage is a benign condition that does not harm the eye.

No treatment is necessary, but you will need to warn the patient that the condition could take weeks to resolve fully. It is worth taking the patient's blood pressure; if the condition is recurrent, check blood coagulation and refer non-urgently to an ophthalmologist.

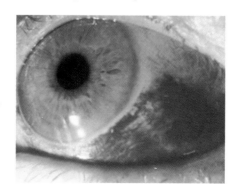

Figure 2.10 Subconjunctival hemorrhage presenting as a patch of bright red blood on the white of the eye.

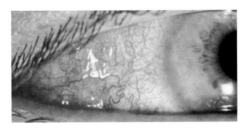

Figure 2.11 Episcleritis presents as a red eye with mild irritation. Redness is often focal rather than diffuse.

Episcleritis (Figure 2.11) presents as a red eye (usually unilateral) with mild irritation, but without the pain associated with scleritis. There is no significant itch or discharge; the redness is more often focal than diffuse. No treatment is necessary unless the redness persists or worsens, in which case referral is appropriate.

Dry eyes are the most common cause of a sensation of dryness, grittiness or burning. Patients may complain of a chronic foreign body sensation – 'There is always something in my eyes'. This disorder is very common among elderly patients, and in younger patients with autoimmune diseases such as rheumatoid arthritis. If severe, it can cause corneal ulceration, but it is usually merely annoying rather than dangerous. The eyes often look completely normal or are mildly red. It is worth trying treatment with lubricating eye drops (artificial tears) every 2 hours, plus a lubricating non-medicated eye ointment at night. Refer routinely if these lubricating treatments do not help.

Blepharitis is chronic, mild inflammation of the eyelids, which often causes secondary eye irritation, burning and foreign body sensation. The eyes themselves may look normal or slightly red. The eyelid margins appear slightly reddened and thickened, often with crusting or matting of the eyelashes (Figure 2.12). Part of the problem is a blockage

Figure 2.12 Blepharitis, presenting as a slightly red eye; the eyelid margins look reddened and thickened, with crusting of the eyelashes.

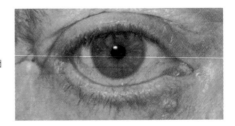

of the eyelids' oil glands, so the patient may find it helpful over the long term to massage the closed eyelids twice daily with a hot, wet face cloth. Gentle cleaning of the eyelid margins, twice daily, with a cotton swab (cotton bud) dipped in diluted 'baby shampoo' may also help to alleviate the symptoms. Patients with blepharitis also often have dry eyes, so prescribe lubricating eye drops as well. Refer routinely if these measures do not help.

Key points – red eye

'Bad' red eye
- If a patient presents with a red eye of unknown cause, with one or more of the 'five Ps' (see page 22), they have a 'bad' red eye.
- Refer all patients with 'bad' red eye *immediately* and *urgently* – emergency treatment can often save the patient's sight.
- Underlying causes of 'bad' red eye include acute glaucoma, iritis, infective corneal ulcer, scleritis and endophthalmitis.

'Good' red eye
- If a patient presents with one or two red eyes, but without pain, photophobia or blurred vision, and the eyes are otherwise normal on examination, they have 'good' red eye/s.
- You can treat these patients yourself; however, they should be referred if they do not begin to improve within 2 weeks, or if their condition worsens.
- Underlying causes of 'good' red eye/s include bacterial, viral and allergic conjunctivitis, subconjunctival hemorrhage, episcleritis, dry eyes and blepharitis.

Treatment
- The only eye drops you should prescribe without an ophthalmologist's opinion are artificial tears, antibiotics (for bacterial conjunctivitis) or mast-cell inhibitors (for allergic conjunctivitis).
- Do not prescribe steroid eye drops without advice from an ophthalmologist, as they can exacerbate infections, and cause cataracts and glaucoma.

The most common causes of blurred vision are refractive error (in the young) and cataract (in the elderly). However, blurred vision can also be the presenting symptom of potentially blinding intraocular disease such as retinal detachment, or potentially fatal extraocular disease such as vasculitis, brain tumor or stroke.

Referral

It is essential to be able to clinically triage your patients with blurred vision into the majority for whom routine written referral to an ophthalmologist is appropriate and the minority who require urgent referral (to be seen the same day). Delay in referral of urgent cases (see below), of even a few days, can cost the patient their sight.

Urgent referral for any patient with blurred vision and one or more of:

- acute or rapidly progressive visual loss
- severe visual loss
- red eye (see Chapter 2) or recent eye trauma (see Chapter 10)
- eye pain
- new-onset flashing lights or floating spots in the vision
- new-onset visual distortion (metamorphopsia)
- a visual field defect (described by the patient or discovered during confrontation field testing)
- RAPD on the swinging light test (see Chapter 1)
- swollen optic disc/s on examination by direct ophthalmoscopy
- symptoms of temporal arteritis (in patients over 50; see page 54)
- diabetes with new-onset visual symptoms (e.g. flashes, floaters)
- transient visual loss not typical of migraine
- any symptoms from which other acute eye or brain disease can be suspected (e.g. new-onset severe headaches).

All children and young adults who present with blurred vision require urgent referral.

Patients with none of the features described opposite may be referred routinely, but should be advised to contact you if there are any major changes in their symptoms while they are waiting to be seen by the ophthalmologist.

Causes of acute visual loss

Patients suspected of having any of the diseases outlined in this section should be referred urgently, as immediate ophthalmic medical or surgical treatment may be able to recover or stabilize sight in some cases.

Retinal detachment. The retina can peel off the back of the eye, usually after traction from the vitreous jelly tears a hole in the retina (Figure 3.1). If the detachment is diagnosed before it reaches the central visual area (the macula), urgent surgical repair can maintain good vision. Short-sighted patients have a greater risk of retinal detachment.

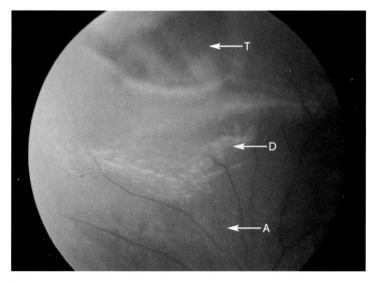

Figure 3.1 Retinal detachment. A, attached retina; D, detached retina; T, tear in retina.

Patients with retinal detachment complain of one or more of:
- flashes – white flashes of light in the peripheral vision
- floaters – new, previously unnoticed, shower of floating spots in the vision
- field loss – a dark 'curtain' or 'cloud' developing over part of the peripheral vision and moving towards the central vision over a period of hours, days or weeks.

Examination shows normal or decreased acuity, sometimes a field defect to confrontation testing and sometimes an RAPD on the swinging light test. The detachment is not usually visible with the direct ophthalmoscope (unless extensive), as its field of view is too small.

Retinal vascular occlusions. One of the branch retinal veins or arteries, or the central retinal vein or artery, become occluded. Vein occlusion is usually due to thrombosis; arterial occlusion is often due to embolism from the carotid artery or heart. Patients complain of sudden or subacute blurring of vision or visual field loss in one eye. Examination shows:
- reduced visual acuity (VA) (although some branch occlusions present with field loss only and no reduction in acuity)
- field defect to confrontation
- RAPD on the swinging light test (sometimes, in severe occlusions).

For arterial occlusions, direct ophthalmoscopy may show retinal pallor and decreased arterial filling in the distribution of the occlusion (sectoral for branch artery occlusion; diffuse with a central macular 'cherry-red spot' in central artery occlusion – Figure 3.2a). However, these signs may easily be missed with the direct ophthalmoscope because of its poor field of view.

Vein occlusions (Figures 3.2b, c) are often more visible on ophthalmoscopy, with sectoral (branch vein) or diffuse (central vein) retinal hemorrhages, tortuous dilated veins and (often) optic disc swelling.

It is important to remember that retinal venous occlusions are often warning signs of previously undetected or undertreated hypertension, diabetes or (in young patients) coagulopathy. Arterial occlusions may be the first sign of temporal arteritis, hypercholesterolemia, hypertension, diabetes, carotid stenosis or a cardiac embolic source (e.g. heart valve disease).

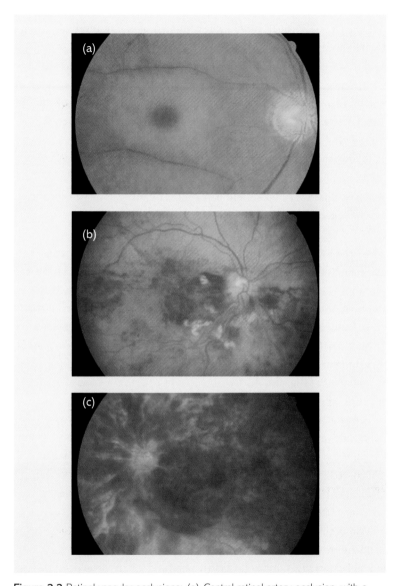

Figure 3.2 Retinal vascular occlusions: (a) Central retinal artery occlusion, with a 'cherry-red spot' due to visible choroidal circulation at the fovea, where the neural retina is very thin and contrasts with the thickened white edematous retina in the surrounding macular area. (b) Hemisphere vein occlusion, with retinal hemorrhages and 'cotton wool spots' confined to the lower half of the retina. (c) Central retinal vein occlusion, with extensive hemorrhages throughout the fundus.

Vitreous hemorrhage is bleeding into the vitreous jelly at the back of the eye (Figure 3.3). Causes include bleeding from abnormal new retinal vessels in proliferative diabetic retinopathy, a retinal tear or detachment, or trauma. Patients complain of floaters and blurred vision. Examination shows normal or reduced acuity, but usually no RAPD unless retinal detachment is also present. The red reflex may be abnormal if there is major hemorrhage. Areas of blood in the vitreous may or may not be visible with the direct ophthalmoscope.

Any diabetic patient complaining of new-onset floaters (with or without blurred vision) should be taken especially seriously, because of the high risk that new vessels are bleeding.

'Wet' age-related macular degeneration (wet ARMD). The macula is the center of the retina and is the area responsible for high-acuity reading vision. Most ARMD is 'dry' (that is, no abnormal new vessels are present) and results in gradually progressive loss of vision.

In 'wet' ARMD, leakage from abnormal new blood vessels (Figure 3.4) causes:
- acute or subacute onset of blurred vision, or sudden worsening of previously poor vision
- distortion of straight lines or shapes (metamorphopsia)
- often, a central blurred or blank spot in the vision, with normal peripheral vision (central scotoma).

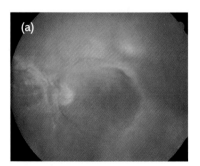 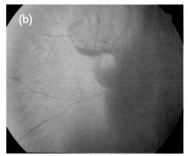

Figure 3.3 Vitreous hemorrhage. (a) Old vitreous hemorrhage in a diabetic patient with fibrovascular proliferations from the disc. The macula is still visible but the peripheral retina is obscured by old hemorrhage. (b) Fresh vitreous hemorrhage partially obscuring the disc.

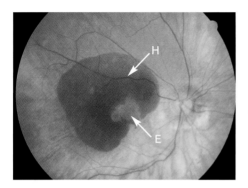

Figure 3.4 Wet age-related macular degeneration, showing central leakage from abnormal new blood vessels. E, elevation formed by new subretinal vessels; H, subretinal hemorrhage.

The macula is very difficult to examine with the direct ophthalmoscope, especially without the use of dilating drops, but it may show hemorrhages and hard exudates. Laser treatment may help to stabilize vision.

Acute optic neuropathy. In this condition, the optic nerve behind one or both eyes loses some or all of its capability to transmit impulses, resulting in blurred vision in the affected eye/s. The cardinal sign in all unilateral optic neuropathies is an RAPD on the swinging light test.

There are many possible causes of acute optic neuropathy. In young adults, the most common cause is 'typical' optic neuritis (an early sign of multiple sclerosis in some, but not all, patients). Rapid unilateral loss of vision occurs, with pain that worsens when the eye moves. The optic disc may appear normal or swollen on ophthalmoscopy (Figure 3.5).

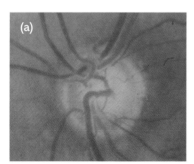
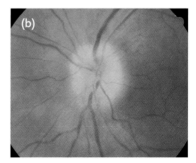

Figure 3.5 Acute optic neuropathy in which the optic disc appears (a) normal or (b) swollen.

In middle-aged or elderly patients, the most common cause is anterior ischemic optic neuropathy – blockage of the fine arteries that supply the optic disc due to temporal arteritis or atherosclerosis. The disease presents as sudden visual loss with a swollen optic disc, which is painless (unless there is a headache associated with temporal arteritis).

Vision loss soon after eye surgery. If the patient develops blurred vision with a 'white' eye soon after eye surgery, they could have retinal detachment, or a swelling of the macula called cystoid macular edema. If they develop blurred vision with a red eye they probably have an infection inside the eyeball (endophthalmitis; see Figure 2.6, page 26).

Causes of gradual visual loss
Patients suspected of having one of the diseases in this section can be referred routinely unless one or more of the criteria for urgent referral are present (e.g. flashes, floaters, visual field defect or RAPD).

Refractive error and presbyopia. It is rare for patients to complain of blurred vision due to uncorrected refractive error, as the first thing patients with blurred vision usually do is have their glasses checked. However, if a patient with gradually progressive blurred vision has not had their glasses prescription reviewed for several years, it is worth arranging this with their optometrist before ophthalmic referral (especially if VA improves with pinhole testing), unless you have found an indication for urgent referral.

The common types of refractive error are:
• myopia (short-sightedness)
• hypermetropia (long-sightedness)
• astigmatism (warped corneal surface)
• presbyopia (the loss of the eye's ability to focus on close objects with age).

Middle-aged patients whose distance vision is fine, but whose reading vision is deteriorating, may be experiencing presbyopia. This is easily corrected with reading glasses or bifocals.

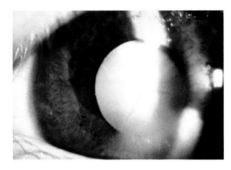

Figure 3.6 The cloudy lens of cataract.

Cataract is a clouding of the eye's normally clear lens (Figure 3.6). Cataract usually occurs in the elderly, or in younger patients with diabetes, intraocular inflammation or eye trauma. Patients complain of gradually progressive blurring of vision, which may be asymmetric, and sometimes of glare in bright lights. Visual fields are full to confrontation, there is no RAPD, the eyes look normal externally (apart from a gray rather than black pupil in cases of advanced cataract) and there may be a dulling of the red reflex.

Cataract extraction and intraocular artificial lens implantation is a common and often highly successful operation, but does entail some risk (approximately 1 in 100 patients develops complications from the procedure).

Chronic glaucoma causes slow, painless loss of vision, which is usually not noticed by the patient because peripheral vision is lost first. Central vision loss signifies severe disease and can occur if the condition is not detected early by routine population screening. Chronic glaucoma is common, and risk increases with age. People with a family history of glaucoma are at increased risk and may develop the disease at a younger age.

Regular glaucoma screening examinations (every 2 years) by an optometrist are recommended for all adults over 40 years of age. The examination should include an eye pressure test and optic disc examination, plus a visual field test if the results of either of these tests are abnormal. Screening may need to begin earlier if there is a family history of glaucoma, or in certain racial groups (e.g. people of African or Caribbean descent).

The eyes of a patient with chronic glaucoma appear entirely normal on examination, apart from raised intraocular pressure (in most but not all patients) and characteristic 'cupping' of one or both optic discs (Figure 3.7). Do not confuse this condition with acute glaucoma, which is much rarer and presents with a painful red eye and blurred vision (see Chapter 2 – red eye).

Eye drops are the usual first-line treatment, but surgery is performed if eye drops fail to control the pressure or if the glaucoma is severe. Be aware that some glaucoma eye drops can have systemic effects; for example, beta-blockers (such as timolol) may exacerbate asthma, bradycardia, depression or hyperlipidemia.

Diabetic maculopathy. All of your practice's diabetic patients should be enrolled for regular (usually annual) diabetic retinopathy screening. The right time to treat diabetic maculopathy (or proliferative retinopathy) with laser is in its early stages, before it becomes symptomatic.

Patients who have advanced diabetic maculopathy that has not been detected by screening complain of blurred vision and metamorphopsia. Early diabetic maculopathy is very difficult to see with the direct ophthalmoscope, particularly without the aid of dilating drops. Advanced cases may show microaneurysms (small red dots) and hard exudates (yellow lipid deposits from leaky microaneurysms) at or near the macula (Figure 3.8).

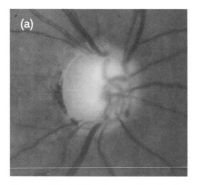 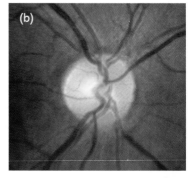

Figure 3.7 (a) The 'cupped' optic disc of chronic glaucoma in which the central cup has expanded to occupy most of the disc. (b) A normal disc, with its small central cup, shown for comparison.

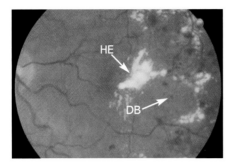

Figure 3.8 An advanced case of diabetic maculopathy, presenting with macular edema and surrounding hard exudates. DB, dot (microaneurysm) and blot hemorrhage; HE, hard exudates.

Because of the high risk of serious retinal disease, diabetic patients who complain of acute or subacute onset of blurred vision or visual distortion require urgent referral.

'Dry' age-related macular degeneration (dry ARMD). In the elderly, age-related changes in the macula often cause gradual, usually mild-to-moderate, loss of vision. The patient complains of increasing difficulty reading and blurred central vision with preserved peripheral vision. The macula is very difficult to examine with the direct ophthalmoscope, especially if dilating drops are not used, but drusen (small yellow spots from the waste products of cell metabolism) or areas of pigment atrophy and/or black pigment clumps may be seen (Figure 3.9).

Superimposed on this gradual decline of vision, a minority of patients also experience a sudden increase in metamorphopsia or a sudden loss of central vision due to the development of wet ARMD.

Low-vision aids, such as magnifiers and good lighting, often help to maximize the patient's vision.

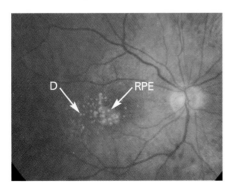

Figure 3.9 Dry age-related macular degeneration. D, drusen (small yellowish deposits in the retina); RPE, atrophy of the retinal pigment epithelium.

Slowly progressive optic neuropathy. Tumors in the orbit or pituitary region often compress one or both optic nerves or the optic chiasm, and usually present with gradual visual field loss and/or loss of VA in one or both eyes.

There are also many other causes of chronic optic neuropathy, including infections, autoimmune disease, pernicious anemia and nutritional deficiency.

A visual field defect (of any type) may be found on confrontation testing, and an RAPD will be found if the condition is unilateral or asymmetric. The optic disc/s may look normal, swollen or, as shown in Figure 3.10, pale. If slowly progressive optic neuropathy is suspected, urgent referral is necessary because there may be an underlying brain tumor.

Gradual loss of vision after cataract surgery. Patients who complain of a slow decline in initially good vision after cataract surgery most commonly have posterior capsular fibrosis (scarring that develops behind the intraocular lens as the eye heals after surgery); this can usually be fixed with laser treatment. Although rare, chronic macular edema and retinal detachment can also occur, as can other eye disease completely unrelated to the cataract surgery.

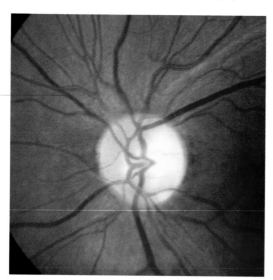

Figure 3.10 Optic disc pallor in a slowly progressive optic neuropathy.

Causes of transient visual loss

Transient visual loss that is not the prodrome of known migraine is always serious and requires urgent ophthalmic referral. Dangerous causes of non-migrainous transient visual loss include carotid stenosis, heart valve disease, transient ischemic attack and papilledema due to a brain tumor.

Transient visual loss in one eye is usually the result of an embolus from a stenosed ipsilateral carotid artery or, less often, an embolus from a cardiac valve. However, in patients over 50, transient visual loss in one eye can also be a warning sign of permanent visual loss from temporal arteritis (urgent treatment at this stage of temporal arteritis can often avert acute bilateral blindness).

Patients with monocular, embolic, transient visual loss (amaurosis fugax) report a sudden loss of vision, as if a curtain comes down over their eye, followed by a spontaneous return of vision a few minutes to an hour later. Eye examination findings after the attack are usually entirely normal.

In some cases, patients may also mistake transient binocular homonymous visual loss (see below) as being in one eye only.

Transient visual loss in both eyes simultaneously is most commonly caused by the binocular 'scintillating scotoma' that occurs before the onset of headache in many patients with migraine. This scotoma may sometimes occur in known migraine patients without headache (acephalgic migraine).

Scintillating scotoma is a homonymous scotoma (a dark area in the same position in each visual field, for example, the left part of the left eye's vision and the left part of the right eye's vision), bordered by zig-zag lines or flashing colored lights. The dark area slowly expands, and then usually disappears as the headache phase of the migraine starts. Scintillating scotomas are also occasionally produced by occipital seizures (including those due to a tumor or vascular malformation).

Transient homonymous field loss or transient bilateral blindness (usually without zig-zags or flashing lights) can also occur in vertebrobasilar transient ischemic attacks, brief episodes of neurological disturbance caused by a reduced blood supply to the occipital lobes.

Papilledema (bilateral optic disc swelling due to raised intracranial pressure) can also cause fading out of vision in one or both eyes, usually for seconds at a time.

Key points – blurred vision

- Most patients with blurred vision have benign, slowly progressive conditions and can be referred routinely to an ophthalmologist. However, blurred vision may also be the first symptom of potentially sight- or life-threatening disease, and patients suspected of having a serious cause of blurred vision must be referred urgently – see referral guide on page 32.
- All people over 40 should be encouraged to have regular glaucoma screenings with their optometrist. Chronic glaucoma is usually asymptomatic until it is very advanced.
- Please check that all your practice's diabetic patients are enrolled for regular eye screening to detect diabetic eye disease. Diabetic retinopathy is best treated at a presymptomatic stage to prevent visual loss.
- Always consider temporal arteritis if a patient over 50 complains of sudden loss of vision or transient blurring of vision.

Referral

The clinical assessment of a patient with double vision (diplopia) is complex, and it is very difficult for non-ophthalmologists to accurately differentiate between serious and non-serious causes. For this reason, all patients with new-onset transient or persisting double vision require urgent referral to an ophthalmologist, ideally to be seen the same day.

All patients with new-onset double vision require urgent referral

Causes of double vision

If a patient has double vision they see two images of a single object. Many adults with double vision have an ischemic third, fourth or sixth nerve palsy, which will usually resolve spontaneously within a few months. However, the fact that a patient has risk factors for an ischemic nerve palsy (such as diabetes or hypertension) is no reassurance that more serious pathology is absent.

New-onset double vision is also a common presenting symptom of potentially fatal brain aneurysms, brain tumors, stroke, myasthenia gravis or temporal arteritis. Brain aneurysms in particular can rupture, killing the patient, within hours of the onset of double vision if they are not immediately diagnosed and treated.

As outlined in the following sections, double vision can result from disease of the orbit, extraocular muscles, neuromuscular junction, ocular motor nerves or brain.

Extraocular muscle or orbit disease. Orbital fractures may cause diplopia by entrapment of, or damage to, the eye muscles.

Thyroid eye disease causes swelling of the extraocular muscles and orbital connective tissue, pushing the eyeball forward (proptosis) and often causing restricted movement of the eye along with diplopia (Figure 4.1).

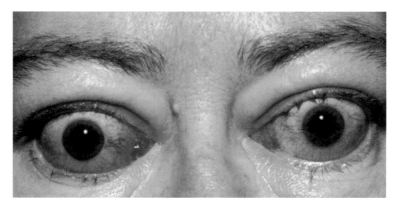

Figure 4.1 Thyroid eye disease, displaying characteristic bilateral proptosis.

The eye muscles are also less commonly affected by infection or autoimmune inflammation of other causes. Orbital tumors may also present with diplopia.

Neuromuscular junction disease (myasthenia) is a relatively common cause of diplopia and/or ptosis (drooping upper eyelid/s) in adults of all ages. Most patients with myasthenia say that their double vision varies from day to day, and is often worst at the end of the day.

Ocular motor nerve palsies. The most common cause of diplopia in patients over 50 is ischemic third, fourth or sixth nerve palsy; this is usually due to diabetes or atherosclerosis, but may also be caused by temporal arteritis.

Third nerve palsy may be partial (affecting one or more of the medial rectus, superior rectus, inferior rectus, inferior oblique or upper-lid levator muscles) or complete (completely paralyzing all these muscles). In either of these presentations, the pupil constrictor muscle, which is also innervated by the third nerve, may be affected (causing a dilated pupil that constricts poorly to light) or unaffected.

Partial third nerve palsy may not be obvious, as it can present as a subtle vertical muscle imbalance (one eye higher than the other) or exotropia (one eye turned out), with horizontal, vertical or oblique double vision.

A complete third nerve palsy presents with a complete ptosis (the eyelid is closed) (Figure 4.2). When the lid is lifted, the eye is seen to be turned out (by the action of the intact sixth nerve on the lateral rectus) and cannot move in any direction except further out towards the ear.

Posterior communicating artery aneurysm causes up to a third of all third nerve palsies (partial or complete). A 'spared' (normal size) or enlarged pupil is *not* a reliable indication of whether an aneurysm is present.

The most common cause overall of third nerve palsy is ischemia.

Fourth nerve palsy causes superior oblique weakness, resulting in hypertropia (i.e. the affected eye is higher than the unaffected eye) and excyclotorsion (outward rotation) of the affected eye, causing vertical and often torsional (tilted) double vision. Eye movements often look normal to casual observation, and special testing is needed for diagnosis.

Fourth nerve palsy may be congenital, and often presents as head tilt in children. For this reason, all children with a head tilt or turn should be seen by an ophthalmologist.

Acquired fourth nerve palsy is often due to blunt head trauma. Adults may present after minor head trauma with rather non-specific visual difficulties and a head tilt. Ischemia is a common cause of fourth nerve palsy. It can also be caused, rarely, by a brain tumor.

Sixth nerve palsy causes lateral rectus weakness with esotropia (the eye is turned in and cannot turn out fully towards the ear), which

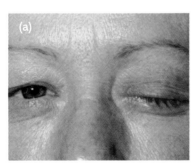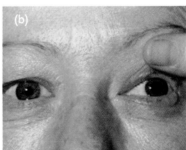

Figure 4.2 Complete third nerve palsy. (a) The patient cannot open the left eye due to complete left ptosis. (b) When the eyelid is lifted the eye is found to be turned out, in this case with a dilated pupil.

results in horizontal double vision (Figure 4.3). Common causes include ischemia (atherosclerosis, diabetes or temporal arteritis) and compression by a brain tumor. Raised intracranial pressure is a less common cause of unilateral or bilateral sixth nerve palsy.

Brain disease. Brain tumors may cause third, fourth or sixth nerve palsy (see above). Brainstem disease such as multiple sclerosis or stroke may cause internuclear ophthalmoplegia, which presents as poor adduction of the eye on the affected side (the eye cannot look fully in towards the nose) and abducting nystagmus of the other eye (the eye develops jerky sideways movements when the patient tries to look out towards the ear).

Disease of higher brain centers can also cause complicated eye movement disorders. For example, brainstem stroke or tumor can cause a vertical eye misalignment (skew deviation), or loss of the ability to look up, down or to one side with both eyes together (gaze palsy).

Temporal arteritis is a sight- and life-threatening disease that only affects patients over 50. It is not uncommon for the patient to complain of intermittent double vision that has disappeared by the time they see a doctor (with a normal eye examination). Alternatively, they may present with a third, fourth or sixth nerve palsy. Urgent referral may save the patient's sight or their life.

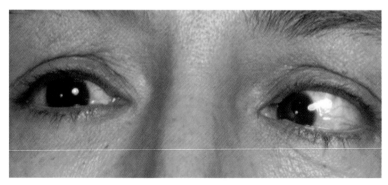

Figure 4.3 Sixth nerve palsy of the right eye, with the patient attempting to look to the right.

Double vision after trauma. Causes of double vision after eye or head trauma include orbital fractures or bruising; third, fourth or sixth nerve palsy due to the initial head trauma or secondary to an expanding intracranial hemorrhage; or brain damage causing an eye movement disorder.

Key points – double vision

- Urgently refer all patients (of any age) with new-onset double vision to an ophthalmologist, ideally to be seen the same day.
- Double vision may be due to disease of the orbit, extraocular muscles, neuromuscular junction, ocular motor nerves or brain. It is often very difficult to accurately diagnose the cause on examination.
- Brain aneurysms – which can be fatal if they are not urgently diagnosed and treated – are a not infrequent cause of double vision in adults; patients often present with partial or complete third nerve palsy. Pupil size is not a reliable indicator of whether an aneurysm is present.
- Overall, the most common cause of diplopia in adults is ischemic third, fourth or sixth nerve palsy.

Red eye, blurred vision and double vision are all common and important eye symptoms. However, you should also listen carefully to the patient for the presence of other symptoms that may indicate serious eye disease.

Referral

> **Urgent referral** for any patient with one or more of:
>
> - flashing lights (other than the visual prodrome of migraine)
> - new-onset floating spots
> - visual field loss (which the patient complains of, or you detect on testing fields to confrontation)
> - visual distortion (metamorphopsia – straight lines look wavy)
> - photophobia (sensitivity to light)
> - pain in the eye (even if vision is normal and the eye is not red)
> - symptoms of temporal arteritis (if the patient is over 50) (see Table 5.2, page 54)

Important symptoms

Flashing lights. Patients with migraine often see flashing or sparkling lights before the onset of their headache; sometimes they experience these symptoms without their usual headache (acephalgic migraine).

Flashing lights that are not the prodrome of migraine are most commonly due to an age change in the vitreous called posterior vitreous detachment, in which the vitreous jelly pulls away from the retina. The resultant minor retinal traction causes retinal neurons to fire, and the patient then sees flashing lights. However, in a minority of patients the flashing lights are caused by major retinal traction resulting in a retinal tear or detachment, which requires urgent laser or surgical treatment.

Floating spots. Most of us, when looking at a blue sky or a white wall, can see small clear or gray floaters in our vision; these are normal imperfections in the vitreous jelly. However, new-onset floaters (gray, black or red spots, cobwebs or blobs) can be due to a retinal tear, retinal detachment or vitreous hemorrhage, and require urgent assessment.

A combination of new-onset floaters and new-onset flashing lights signals a higher likelihood of a retinal tear or detachment.

Visual field loss. Table 5.1 outlines the different types of visual field defect in terms of how they are perceived by the patient, the anatomic site at which they occur and the causes of each type of defect.

TABLE 5.1

Types of visual field defect

Visual field defect*	Anatomic site	Common causes
Right homonymous hemianopia		
  L R	Left retrochiasmal visual pathway (optic tract, lateral geniculate nucleus, optic radiation, occipital visual cortex)	Stroke, brain tumor, head trauma
Bitemporal hemianopia		
  L R	Optic chiasm	Compression by pituitary tumor
Any other field defects (unilateral or bilateral)		
	Retina or optic nerve	Unilateral or bilateral macular, retinal or optic nerve disease of any cause

*Drawn as the patient would see them. L, left eye; R, right eye.

Persisting visual field loss is always due to serious eye, optic nerve or brain disease. Some patients will spontaneously mention that their vision is bad only in a certain area (e.g. only out to the side) in one or both eyes. Others will realize (if you ask them) that their blurred vision is only in part of the visual field (Figure 5.1), and some patients may be asymptomatic and the field defect only noted on examination.

Causes include retinal disease, optic nerve disease, a pituitary tumor compressing the intracranial optic nerve/s or chiasm, and retrochiasmal stroke or brain tumor.

Transient visual field loss. Transient binocular homonymous field loss may occur as part of the migraine prodrome. This is usually a slowly expanding visual field defect surrounded by flashing lights or

(a)   (b)

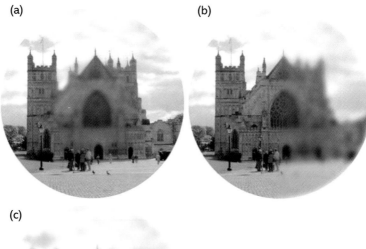

(c)

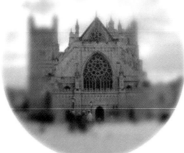

Figure 5.1 Simulation of visual field loss, as seen by a patient with one eye (other eye covered): (a) central scotoma; (b) temporal hemifield loss; (c) peripheral field loss.

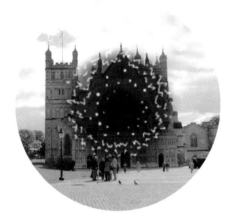

Figure 5.2 Simulation of what a patient sees as a visual prodrome to migraine: an expanding, scintillating scotoma.

zig-zag lines (a scintillating scotoma) (Figure 5.2). Transient homonymous visual field loss (usually without flashing lights) may also occur in vertebrobasilar transient ischemic attacks (TIAs).

Visual distortion (metamorphopsia) is almost always a symptom of macular (central retinal) disease (Figure 5.3). If onset is sudden in elderly patients, it may be a warning sign of wet age-related macular degeneration (ARMD). There are also many other macular diseases.

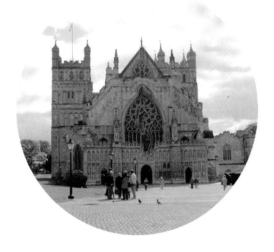

Figure 5.3 Simulation of metamorphopsia (visual distortion).

Photophobia (sensitivity to light) can be the earliest symptom of iritis, before the eye becomes red or the vision becomes blurred.

It is also important to check for non-ocular causes of photophobia (e.g. meningitis).

Eye pain or eye ache can occur in early acute glaucoma, scleritis or iritis, before the eye becomes red.

Pain may also be referred to the eye from intracranial structures (e.g. those compressed by a brain tumor), and common headaches or trigeminal neuralgia can also result in eye pain.

Temporal arteritis (giant cell arteritis) is a treatable but acutely sight- and life-threatening disease that only affects patients over the age of 50. It is therefore important to ask any patient over 50 who has headaches or visual symptoms specifically whether they have any of the symptoms of temporal arteritis described in Table 5.2.

TABLE 5.2

Symptoms of temporal arteritis

Visual symptoms

Transient visual loss in one or both eye/s

Acute persisting visual loss in one or both eye/s

Transient or permanent double vision

Headaches

New type of headache (not previously experienced by the patient); often non-specific and not necessarily temporal

Other symptoms

Jaw claudication (ache in the jaw muscles after chewing; resolves with rest)

Scalp tenderness (to touch or on brushing the hair)

Tongue, ear or neck pain

Myalgias (many patients with polymyalgia rheumatica also develop temporal arteritis, and vice versa)

Weight loss, fevers, night sweats, fatigue

The only clinical sign of temporal arteritis (other than signs of its complications) is tenderness and/or non-pulsatility of the temporal arteries on palpation; however, this is often unreliable. Blood tests usually reveal an elevated erythrocyte sedimentation rate (ESR) and C-reactive protein (CRP) level.

Even if no visual symptoms are present initially, patients with untreated temporal arteritis can suddenly go permanently blind in one or both eyes, usually from anterior ischemic optic neuropathy. If, however, the disease is suspected early, and the patient is referred urgently and is treated with high-dose steroids, visual loss and life-threatening complications can usually be prevented.

Key points – other important symptoms

- Patients with any of the following symptoms require urgent ophthalmic referral:
  - flashing lights (other than the visual prodrome of migraine)
  - new-onset floating spots
  - visual field loss
  - visual distortion
  - photophobia (sensitivity to light)
  - pain in the eye (even if vision is normal and the eye is not red)
  - symptoms of temporal arteritis (if the patient is over 50)
- A combination of flashing lights and floating spots may indicate a retinal tear or detachment.
- Visual distortion is almost always a symptom of serious macular disease.
- Photophobia or eye pain may indicate early iritis or acute glaucoma.
- Urgent referral of patients with symptoms of temporal arteritis could save their sight or their life.

Gritty, itchy or watery eyes are very common complaints, and in general are annoying to the patient rather than dangerous.

Referral

Routine referral is appropriate for patients with gritty, itchy or watery eyes if their discomfort persists or worsens. Patients with these symptoms do not require urgent referral, unless you discover another abnormality when taking a history or during examination.

> Refer routinely if the discomfort persists or worsens.

Gritty eyes or foreign body sensation

If a patient complains 'there is something in my eye' (foreign body sensation), they may well have a foreign body on the cornea (see Chapter 10 – eye trauma) or conjunctiva, or between the upper or lower eyelid and the eyeball. If a foreign body is not visible, remember to evert the upper lid (see Chapter 1 – eye examination) and look for a foreign body under the lid.

Be aware that a dendritic corneal ulcer, which is caused by the herpes simplex virus (HSV), may present as a gritty eye rather than a red, painful eye, because the virus makes the cornea partially numb. However, the patient will often complain of blurred vision and will have mildly reduced visual acuity; corneal examination with fluorescein and blue light will usually reveal the ulcer.

Other causes of gritty eyes include small corneal ulcers of other causes (non-infectious ulcers such as marginal keratitis or early infectious ulcers), corneal abrasions, dry eye, blepharitis, inturned eyelashes, and ectropion or entropion.

Dry eye may cause a slightly red eye, or the patient may have normal-looking eyes. Corneal abnormalities caused by dry eye are only visible on slit-lamp examination. Dry eye should be suspected if the patient complains that their eyes feel 'dry' or 'burning', or if the sensation worsens during reading (due to the decreased blink rate we all have while reading). Prescribe artificial tears to be administered frequently (every 2 hours) and then reduce the frequency as the symptoms improve. Refer routinely if the eye drops do not help.

Blepharitis is a chronic inflammation of the eyelid margins that can occur at any age. Patients commonly complain of chronic eye irritation, grittiness and itching. Patients with blepharitis are also predisposed to the development of chalazia (eyelid lumps caused by inflammation of the oil glands; see page 78) and marginal keratitis (small peripheral corneal ulcers).

Initially, tell the patient to treat the condition with hot compresses to the eyelids (use a warm face cloth) and to clean the eyelid margins carefully with a cotton swab (cotton bud) dipped in diluted baby shampoo twice daily (lid scrubs). You must warn the patient that these measures may take several months before they start to alleviate the symptoms and may need to be continued indefinitely. Refer routinely if there is no improvement.

Inturned eyelashes can be removed with fine forceps. However, patients with recurrent inturned lashes should be referred for more permanent treatment.

Ectropion and entropion (outward or inward rolling of the lower eyelid, respectively) can both present with foreign body sensation. Eye irritation occurs in ectropion because the outward drooping lid exposes the eye, while in entropion the inturned lid's lashes abrade the cornea. Surgical treatment is possible.

Itchy eyes

Eye itch without redness is most commonly due to allergic conjunctivitis; however, mild itching may also be caused by dry eye or blepharitis. If allergic conjunctivitis is suspected, topical mast-cell inhibitor eye drops (such as sodium cromoglycate) may be tried. Refer routinely if the eye

drops don't alleviate the symptoms. Steroid treatment gives relief but
should only be used under close ophthalmic supervison, and only in the
short term, as it can cause glaucoma and cataracts.

Watery eyes (epiphora)

The patient complains of constant or intermittent 'tears in the eyes',
which sometimes stream down the cheeks and require frequent eye
wiping, without eye redness, pain or irritation. In adults, watery eyes
are usually due to age-related blockage of the nasolacrimal ducts, or to
ectropion, both of which can be corrected with surgery.

Key points – gritty, itchy or watery eyes

- Most patients with gritty, itchy or watery eyes do not need
  urgent referral, unless serious abnormalities are found when
  taking a history or on examination. You can treat many patients
  with these conditions yourself, as described in the chapter.
- It is important to use a blue light and fluorescein drops to
  examine the cornea, as occasionally a viral dendritic corneal
  ulcer will present with a gritty or irritated eye (no pain is felt
  because the virus makes the eye numb).
- Remember to evert the upper eyelid in patients complaining of
  a 'gritty' feeling or foreign body sensation, to look for a foreign
  body under the lid.

Patients will sometimes have no problems with their vision, but will present with concerns about an eye abnormality that they, their family or their optician has seen. Alternatively, you might notice an abnormality in the eyes of an asymptomatic patient.

Referral

Many abnormalities of eye appearance are minor and of no consequence; however, some abnormalities herald serious disease and require urgent referral, ideally to be seen on the same day.

Urgent referral for any patient with one or more of:

- acute red eye/s with proptosis (forward movement of the eye/s)
- bilateral optic disc swelling (seen on ophthalmoscopy)
- unequal pupils plus double vision
- an abnormal (dull or white) red reflex and/or white pupil
- new-onset nystagmus (constant eye movement); however, if the patient has other neurological symptoms they should be referred to a neurologist instead of an ophthalmologist

Semi-urgent referral for any patient with one or more of:

- unequal pupils that have not previously been noted
- subacute or gradual-onset proptosis
- pale optic disc/s (seen on ophthalmoscopy) or any other serious abnormality (e.g. signs of advanced diabetic retinopathy) that has not previously been noted by an ophthalmologist, when the patient is otherwise asymptomatic

---

Routine referral. Other patients with abnormal eye appearance may be referred routinely, unless other serious abnormalities are found when taking a history or during your eye examination.

Proptosis

Proptosis is a condition in which one or both eyes become pushed forwards due to enlargement of the orbital contents, vascular engorgement or an orbital tumor (Figure 7.1). Causes of acute proptosis with a red eye include orbital cellulitis, autoimmune orbital inflammation and carotid–cavernous fistula. Subacute or gradually progressive unilateral or bilateral proptosis with red eye/s is most commonly caused by thyroid eye disease (associated with Graves' disease). Orbital tumors usually present with gradually progressive proptosis of one eye without redness.

Orbital cellulitis is a bacterial (or occasionally fungal) infection of the orbital soft tissue, which usually spreads to the orbit having started as ethmoid sinusitis (inflammation of the ethmoid paranasal sinus, which forms part of the nasal wall of the orbit). Patients complain of pain and sometimes double vision or blurred vision. Examination usually shows fever, red eye, mild to severe proptosis and often limited eye movements (Figure 7.2) (see pages 72–3). Secondary meningitis or encephalitis can occur, so this is a life-threatening disease that requires urgent admission.

Autoimmune orbital inflammation closely mimics orbital cellulitis in almost all respects, except that usually there is no fever and onset may be less acute.

Carotid–cavernous fistula is an abnormal communication between the carotid arterial system and the venous cavernous sinus. High-pressure arterial blood from the internal carotid artery flows into the cavernous

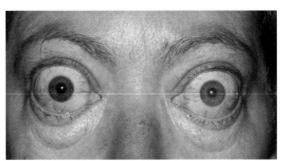

Figure 7.1 Bilateral proptosis due to longstanding thyroid eye disease.

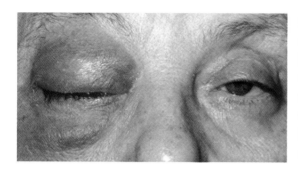

Figure 7.2 Orbital cellulitis – acute infection of the tissues immediately surrounding the eye, with noticeable lid edema and redness.

sinus and then forwards into the orbit. If severe, this sometimes results in pulsatile proptosis in which the eye can be seen and/or felt to move forwards in time with the pulse.

Thyroid eye disease is the most common cause of proptosis in adults, and usually has a subacute or gradual onset. The eyes' appearance can range from slightly red to very red with severe conjunctival swelling. The condition usually occurs in association with Graves' disease (idiopathic hyperthyroidism). The course of the eye disease has no relation to the course of the hyperthyroidism (it may occur before, during or after the patient's hyperthyroid period), and treatment of the hyperthyroidism has no effect on the eye disease.

Thyroid eye disease is not usually a dangerous eye condition, but it can be very annoying for patients who can suffer:
- cosmetic embarrassment due to their eye appearance
- gritty, watering, irritable eyes
- double vision due to tightening of the swollen extraocular muscles.

However, sight-threatening complications can sometimes occur: the corneas can become ulcerated in association with severe proptosis if the eyelids cannot be fully closed; and compressive optic neuropathy, in which the optic nerve is squeezed by the enlarged extraocular muscles, can result in permanent loss of vision.

Orbital tumors. Tumors of many kinds may present with proptosis at any age. Orbital tumors may present with a proptosed but otherwise normal-appearing eye or, less commonly, they may mimic orbital cellulitis (acute red eye with proptosis).

Abnormal optic disc/s

Sometimes you will discover an abnormal optic disc on ophthalmoscopy, despite the fact that the patient has not complained of eye problems. The optic discs are the only visible part of the brain, and as such a change in their appearance can herald significant intracranial disease.

Swollen disc/s. The optic discs are normally flat and pink, with a paler central 'cup'. When the intracranial pressure is raised significantly (due to tumor, hemorrhage or hydrocephalus) both optic discs swell (papilledema) (Figure 7.3). The brain's subarachnoid space normally extends forwards around the optic nerves. If intracranial pressure is raised the high-pressure cerebrospinal fluid squeezes both nerves, causing disc swelling.

Both optic discs are usually obviously swollen if intracranial pressure is very high, but in less severe cases disc swelling may be mild and subtle, asymmetric or even unilateral. The absence of disc swelling does not exclude raised intracranial pressure.

It is also possible for unilateral or bilateral disc swelling to occur with normal intracranial pressure, as a result of unilateral or bilateral optic nerve disease of any cause (e.g. inflammation, ischemia or infiltration with tumor).

> It is important that you perform ophthalmoscopy, looking for optic disc swelling, on all patients who complain of headache. Bilateral disc swelling may be the first and only sign of a brain tumor.

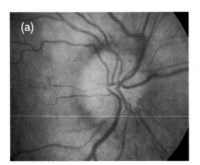 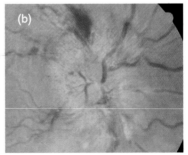

Figure 7.3 Optic disc swelling: (a) moderate; (b) severe.

Disc swelling can be seen in central retinal vein occlusion but will have associated hemorrhages at the disc and in the retina.

Pale disc/s. Ongoing or previous damage to optic nerve axons causes the optic disc/s to appear pale (Figure 7.4a); if this is advanced it is called optic atrophy. Patients with disc pallor usually complain of blurred vision or field loss; however, occasionally it is detected incidentally. Ongoing compression of the optic nerves or chiasm by a tumor is a relatively common cause of optic disc pallor.

Cupped disc/s. By far the most common cause of a cupped disc (expansion of the normally fairly small central cup) is chronic glaucoma (Figure 7.4b). This disease is usually asymptomatic until advanced, because it causes a slow decrease in peripheral vision long before the patient notices central blurring. Chronic glaucoma is most commonly detected on routine screening.

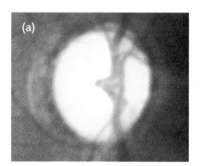 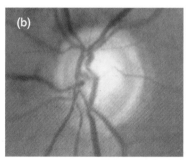

Figure 7.4 (a) Pale optic disc. (b) Cupped optic disc of chronic glaucoma.

Unequal pupils

Sometimes a patient is noted to have different-sized pupils. The chance of serious disease is low if all of the following are present:
- the patient is asymptomatic
- there is no eye redness, blurred vision, double vision, ptosis, pain or headache
- there is no history of cancer
- there is no history of head or neck trauma.

The common causes of unequal pupils are detailed overleaf.

Physiological anisocoria. One-fifth of healthy people have a slight but visible difference in pupil size between the two eyes. They are completely asymptomatic, and have no ptosis or other abnormalities.

Iris disease. The second most common cause of unequal pupil size is previous eye disease, trauma or operation. Mechanical damage to the iris caused by these events may result in a pupil that is smaller or larger than normal, or that has a distorted rather than circular shape.

Third nerve palsy. It is very rare for partial third nerve palsy from a tumor or aneurysm to cause an enlarged pupil in isolation (without double vision, ptosis or a visible abnormality of eye movement).

The presence of an enlarged pupil in a patient with double vision from partial third nerve palsy indicates a high risk of serious underlying disease such as nerve compression by an aneurysm.

Horner's syndrome is the combination of miosis (a smaller than usual pupil) and slight ptosis (a drooping upper lid) on the same side (Figure 7.5). Both of these signs can be subtle and are easily missed. Horner's syndrome occurs as a result of damage to the sympathetic nerve supply to the eye and eyelid; it may be caused by disease in the brainstem, cervical spinal cord, brachial plexus, lung apex, neck, base of skull or cavernous sinus. Such diseases include internal carotid artery dissection (spontaneous or following head or neck trauma), apical lung tumor (Pancoast syndrome) and tumors of the brain, skull base or neck; however, in many cases no cause is identified.

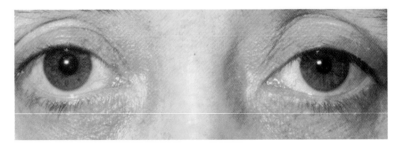

Figure 7.5 Left Horner's syndrome. The patient has a smaller pupil and slightly drooping upper lid on the left-hand side.

Adie's tonic pupil is a benign condition in which one pupil is enlarged (rarely both pupils), without ptosis or diplopia. Patients may complain of blurred vision, because they lose the ability to focus on near objects. The affected pupil shows sluggish or absent constriction to a bright light, but still constricts slowly when the patient is asked to focus on a near object (known as light-near dissociation). The patient may also have depressed limb tendon reflexes of unknown cause.

Abnormal red reflex and/or white pupils

Normally, a patient's pupils look black on casual observation. Red reflex examination by direct ophthalmoscopy will produce a diffuse red or orange glow that fills the pupils; this is the reflection from the back of the eye seen through the ophthalmoscope in a dark room (the cause of 'red eye' in flash photographs).

Red reflex examination is an essential part of every neonate's initial examination after birth. If a child's red reflex is noted to be dark, absent or white (Figure 7.6), on one or both sides, a life-threatening retinoblastoma or sight-threatening congenital cataract could be present.

An abnormal red reflex is not as important a sign in adults, but can be seen in patients with advanced cataract, severe vitreous hemorrhage or advanced retinal detachment.

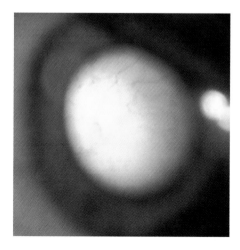

Figure 7.6 A white pupil due to retinoblastoma.

Nystagmus (constant eye movement)

Nystagmus is an uncontrollable, repetitive eye movement that usually affects both eyes. The movement may be horizontal (side to side), vertical (up and down), rotational or a combination of all these types. Causes include:

- poor vision in both eyes from early childhood (due to retinal or optic nerve disease, or congenital cataracts)
- a congenital motor control abnormality of the eyes, with an otherwise normal visual pathway and a normal brain function (congenital idiopathic nystagmus)
- congenital or acquired brainstem or cerebellar disease (tumor, stroke, multiple sclerosis, metabolic disease)
- middle-ear disease (e.g. Ménière's disease)
- drug-related side effects.

Diabetic retinopathy

Regular retinal screening of your diabetic patients by an ophthalmologist or via an accredited retinal screening service is essential for picking up the signs of early maculopathy or proliferative retinopathy. If detected early, the progression of both of these diseases can usually be halted with laser treatment, and the patient's sight can be saved.

> **Make sure that every patient with diabetes in your practice is booked for regular retinal screening.**

The best time to detect and treat serious diabetic retinopathy is *before* the patient develops blurred vision.

The early stages of diabetic maculopathy and retinopathy may be very difficult or impossible to see with the direct ophthalmoscope, but if you are examining for retinopathy in your adult diabetic patients, ophthalmoscopy is much more accurate if you first dilate their pupils with tropicamide 1%. The early stages of diabetic maculopathy and retinopathy are best detected by slit-lamp fundus-lens examination.

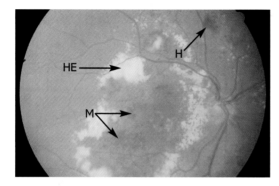

Figure 7.7 Advanced diabetic maculopathy. H, hemorrhage; HE, hard exudates (yellow deposits); M, microaneurysms.

Diabetic maculopathy often consists, in the early stages, of a few microaneurysms (small red dots) and subtle retinal edema. Advanced diabetic maculopathy may show microaneurysms, hemorrhages, hard exudates (yellow deposits) and major swelling of the macular retina (Figure 7.7).

Non-proliferative diabetic retinopathy. Mild-to-moderate non-proliferative retinopathy (previously called 'background' diabetic retinopathy) consists of scattered microaneurysms and hemorrhages, and, in some cases, hard exudates.

Severe non-proliferative diabetic retinopathy (previously called 'preproliferative' retinopathy) provides additional warning signs that proliferative changes are likely within the next year (Figure 7.8). These include tortuosity and variable caliber (beading) of the retinal veins, widespread hemorrhages and cotton-wool spots (small fluffy white areas, previously called soft exudates).

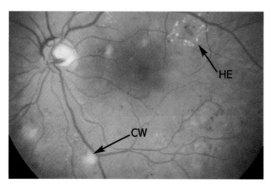

Figure 7.8 Non-proliferative diabetic retinopathy, displaying hemorrhages and cotton-wool spots (small, fluffy white areas). CW, cotton-wool spot; HE, ring of hard exudate.

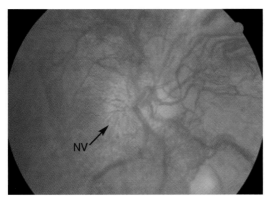

Figure 7.9 Proliferative diabetic retinopathy – abnormal new blood vessels growing from the retina into the vitreous jelly. NV, extensive new disc vessels.

Proliferative diabetic retinopathy. Abnormal new blood vessels grow from the optic disc or retina into the vitreous jelly (Figure 7.9), and can cause blindness from severe vitreous hemorrhage or by causing traction retinal detachment.

Hypertensive retinopathy

Hypertensive patients do not require specific eye screening for this condition in the way that diabetic patients do. Although the presence of hypertensive retinopathy is a useful indication that marked hypertension has been present for some time, it does not usually cause vision problems in itself. The only time hypertensive retinopathy causes visual symptoms is in cases of acute malignant hypertension, when severe bilateral disc swelling and macular edema may occur.

Changes seen in mild-to-moderate hypertensive retinopathy include narrowing of the retinal arterioles and arteriovenous nipping, in which the retinal veins are focally narrowed where they are crossed by sclerosed arteries (Figure 7.10). Changes due to severe malignant hypertension include disc swelling, retinal hemorrhages, hard exudates and macular edema.

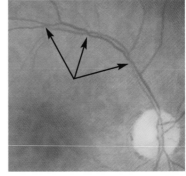

Figure 7.10 Hypertensive retinopathy with arteriovenous nipping (arrowed).

Abnormal spot on the eye surface

Patients or their relatives occasionally notice a spot on the surface of the eye. Common causes for this include:

- pingueculum (a small, yellowish lump medial to the cornea) (Figure 7.11)
- pterygium (a 'wing' of clear or pink tissue growing from the medial conjunctiva onto the adjacent cornea) (Figure 7.12)
- conjunctival nevus (a brown spot on the conjunctiva) (Figure 7.13).

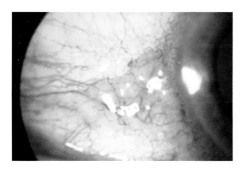

Figure 7.11 Pingueculum – a small, yellowish lump medial to the cornea.

Figure 7.12 Pterygium – a thickened, triangular layer of tissue growing from the conjunctiva onto the adjacent cornea.

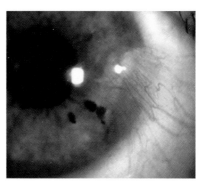

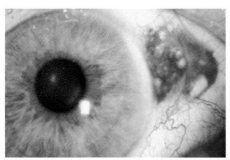

Figure 7.13 Conjunctival nevus – a brown spot on the conjunctiva.

Malignant ocular surface lesions are rare, but occur more often in the elderly.

Patients with newly noticed eye surface spots should be referred for an ophthalmic opinion; routine referral is adequate unless there is particular suspicion of malignancy.

Key points – abnormal eye appearance

- Urgently refer patients who present with any of the following signs:
  - acute red eye with proptosis (forward movement of one or both eyes) (possible orbital cellulitis)
  - bilateral optic disc swelling (possible papilledema from brain tumor)
  - unequal pupils plus double vision (possible partial third nerve palsy from aneurysm)
  - an abnormal (dull or white) red reflex and/or white pupil in children (possible retinoblastoma or congenital cataract)
  - new-onset nystagmus (associated neurological symptoms usually mandate urgent referral to a neurologist rather than an ophthalmologist).
- Asymptomatic patients with unequal pupils that have not been previously noted, gradual-onset proptosis or pale optic discs should be referred semi-urgently.
- It is very important to perform ophthalmoscopy, looking for optic disc swelling, on all patients who complain of headache; bilateral disc swelling may be the first and only sign of a brain tumor.
- Remember to ensure that all your diabetic patients are enrolled for regular retinal screening examinations – these can save their sight.

Diseases of the eyelids are most commonly age-related abnormalities of eyelid position, or benign eyelid lumps. Rarely, however, serious disease can present as an eyelid abnormality.

Referral

Urgent referral is required for one or more of:

- acute unilateral/bilateral eyelid swelling with red eye and proptosis
- any of the signs of orbital cellulitis (see page 72)
- preseptal cellulitis in a child, or in an adult if it does not settle with the use of oral antibiotics
- acute onset of unilateral or bilateral ptosis with double vision, unequal pupils, arm or leg muscle weakness or problems with breathing or swallowing
- herpes zoster ophthalmicus (shingles around the eye)
- new-onset seventh nerve palsy of any cause

Semi-urgent referral for any patient with:

- suspected eyelid skin cancer
- entropion with eyelashes abrading the cornea

You can treat patients with the following conditions yourself, but refer them if the problem persists or worsens:

- stye
- chalazion
- preseptal cellulitis (in a non-febrile adult)
- blepharitis.

Routine referral is appropriate for patients with other eyelid problems (e.g. ectropion).

Eyelid redness and swelling

It is essential to differentiate orbital cellulitis from preseptal cellulitis. Orbital cellulitis is a sight- and life-threatening infection of the deep soft tissues of the orbit around and behind the eye. By contrast, preseptal cellulitis is an infection of the eyelid skin, and is harmless provided it does not progress to orbital cellulitis. Fortunately, it is usually possible to make the distinction between the two conditions on clinical grounds.

Orbital cellulitis. A patient with eyelid redness and swelling plus one or more of the signs shown in Table 8.1 has orbital cellulitis (Figure 8.1) until proven otherwise.

TABLE 8.1

Critical symptoms and signs of orbital cellulitis

Eyelid redness and swelling, plus one or more of:

- Fever
- Pain
- Double vision
- Blurred vision
- A red eye
- Proptosis
- Restricted eye movement in any direction
- Sluggish pupil or relative afferent pupillary defect (RAPD)

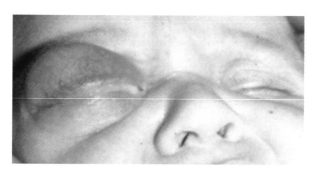

Figure 8.1
Orbital
cellulitis.

Patients with suspected orbital cellulitis require urgent admission for intravenous antibiotics (and sometimes surgery). Orbital cellulitis may be mimicked by several other conditions, all of which are also serious (e.g. carotid–cavernous fistula).

Preseptal cellulitis usually starts with an infected pimple or stye. None of the symptoms or signs of orbital cellulitis already described is present, and although there is localized eyelid redness and swelling (Figure 8.2) the patient is otherwise well and the eye looks normal on lifting the lid.

Children with preseptal cellulitis and adults with preseptal cellulitis and fever are usually admitted for intravenous antibiotic treatment (because of the risk of septicemia or progression to orbital cellulitis). Non-febrile adults who are otherwise well can usually be safely treated with oral antibiotics by their primary care physician, unless the infection worsens or persists. Broad-spectrum oral antibiotics such as flucloxacillin plus amoxicillin–clavulanic acid are often first-line treatment.

Eyelid swelling (edema) without redness can occur in allergic reactions, anaphylactic reactions and nephrotic syndrome. Mild allergic reactions are treated with oral antihistamines. Patients with anaphylactic reactions or nephrotic syndrome require urgent care from the relevant specialist physicians.

Eyelid redness without swelling, in which the eyelid margins are red but without any marked eyelid swelling, is most commonly caused by chronic blepharitis (see pages 30–1 and 57).

Figure 8.2 Preseptal cellulitis with localized eyelid redness and swelling.

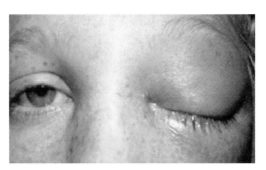

Abnormal eyelid position or function

Lid retraction, in which the upper eyelid is too high, occurs most commonly as a result of thyroid eye disease (see Chapter 7 – abnormal eye appearance). Lid retraction gives a 'staring' appearance to the affected eye/s, and is usually more of a cosmetic embarrassment than a dangerous problem. Corrective surgery is possible.

Ptosis, in which the upper eyelid is too low ('drooping' upper lid; Figure 8.3), has a number of serious causes, including myasthenia, Horner's syndrome and third nerve palsy. However, the most common cause in middle-aged or elderly patients is age-related ptosis due to weakening of the levator muscle's insertion in the upper eyelid (aponeurotic ptosis). In adults with ptosis, the prime concern is to exclude any serious underlying cause; once this has been achieved surgical correction is usually very successful.

Rarely, children are born with a unilateral or bilateral congenital ptosis; these children should be semi-urgently referred as the drooping lid/s can prevent normal visual development.

Ectropion, in which the lower eyelid is turned out, is most commonly due to age-related degeneration and stretching of the eyelid tissues (Figure 8.4); however, rarely, the condition can be due to seventh nerve palsy or scarring. The lower lid hangs away from the eye and can

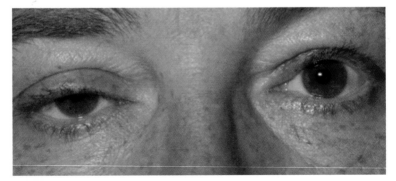

Figure 8.3 Ptosis, a drooping of the upper eyelid. The patient in this figure has an untreated congenital ptosis, but the disorder is usually age related or due to third nerve palsy, myasthenia or Horner's syndrome (see page 64).

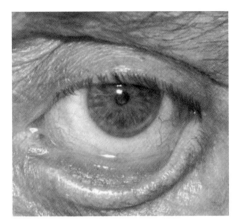

Figure 8.4 Ectropion – the lower eyelid is turned out from the eye, causing irritation and watering.

cause chronic irritation and watering. Patients with ectropion should be referred routinely for corrective surgery, which is usually very successful.

Entropion, in which the lower eyelid is turned in, is also usually due to age-related changes in the lid (Figure 8.5). The lower eyelid rolls inwards, which sometimes causes the eyelashes to abrade the cornea and create foreign body sensation. If severe, this can cause a corneal ulcer.

Patients with entropion should be referred urgently if a corneal abrasion or ulcer is present; otherwise routine referral for corrective surgery is appropriate.

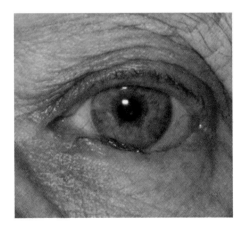

Figure 8.5 Entropion – the lower eyelid is turned inwards, causing the eyelashes to abrade the cornea.

Seventh nerve palsy, whether idiopathic or of known cause (tumor, infection, inflammation, traumatic, postsurgical), can result in decreased orbicularis muscle function and poor eyelid closure (Figure 8.6).

Patients with seventh nerve palsy need to be seen urgently by an ophthalmologist (not referred routinely), as all patients with poor lid closure are at high risk of developing an exposure corneal ulcer.

Blepharospasm is an intermittent or constant eyelid spasm that results in too much eyelid closure. If on one side only, the condition is usually associated with lower facial spasm on the same side (hemifacial spasm); or spasm can occur bilaterally without lower facial involvement (bilateral blepharospasm).

All these patients should see an ophthalmologist to rule out an ocular or neurological cause for the spasm. Many patients then benefit from botulinum toxin injections to relax the contracting muscles.

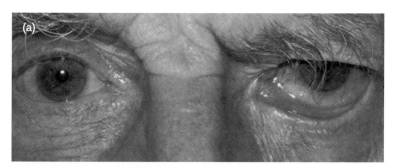

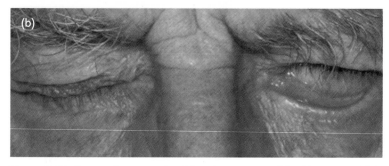

Figure 8.6 Left seventh nerve palsy: (a) with eyes open; (b) with attempted lid closure – full closure is not possible on the affected side.

Skin rashes around the eye

The skin around the eyes is susceptible to most rashes that can occur elsewhere on the skin. However, two of the most common periocular rashes are herpes zoster ophthalmicus (shingles around the eye) and contact allergic rashes.

Herpes zoster ophthalmicus (HZO) is caused by the varicella zoster virus and presents as shingles in the distribution of the ophthalmic division of the trigeminal nerve (V1). A vesicular rash (often severe) appears on half the forehead and scalp; the rash sometimes extends down the midline of the nose and sometimes affects the eyelids (Figure 8.7). Any of these patients can also develop involvement of the eyeball itself, with corneal ulcers, iritis and optic nerve or orbital complications, and therefore all need to be seen by an ophthalmologist.

It is important that all these patients begin a course of oral anti-varicella zoster virus treatment (e.g. aciclovir or valaciclovir) immediately after they have seen you, as this shortens the course of the disease and reduces the risk of serious eye complications. Neuralgic pain, which may be persistent and severe, is common after the rash resolves.

Other periorbital rashes. Patients may develop contact allergic rashes to eye drops or makeup. Generalized skin disease (e.g. atopic eczema) may also involve the periorbital area.

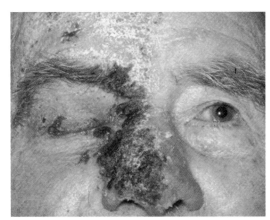

Figure 8.7 Herpes zoster ophthalmicus.

Eyelid lumps

Inflammatory lumps usually have a fairly rapid onset, are usually red and/or tender, and may fluctuate in size over several days or weeks. Tumors, on the other hand, usually grow gradually and are usually not red or tender. Any type of skin tumor can develop in the eyelid skin; you should suspect a malignant tumor if a lid lump progressively enlarges, changes in appearance or causes loss of eyelashes.

Inflammatory lumps

A chalazion is a small, non-infectious, inflammatory mass that originates from blocked meibomian oil glands in the upper or lower eyelid. It may present as a red, tender swelling or a painless, non-tender lump deep in the eyelid tissue (Figure 8.8).

Chalazia are usually associated with blepharitis, which should be treated. These lumps almost always go away with time, but if they are large and persistent they can be surgically treated. Surgery is not usually performed on children, unless the lump is very large, because a general anesthetic is required; in adults it is a simple procedure carried out under local anesthetic. Do not prescribe antibiotic drops or tablets; these treatments will not work, as the lesion is not infected.

A stye is a small, pimple-like infection that may develop around the base of an eyelash (Figure 8.9). Removal of the offending lash may cure the problem. If localized skin redness occurs a short course of oral antibiotics may be given.

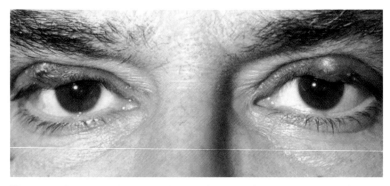

Figure 8.8 Bilateral chalazia – small, non-infectious, inflammatory masses of the eyelids.

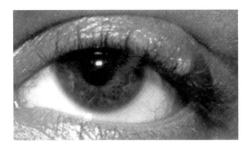

Figure 8.9 Stye – small, pimple-like infection at the base of an eyelash.

Eyelid abscess. Occasionally a small lid lesion may progress to an eyelid abscess, which is a tense, tender cystic swelling, often with surrounding preseptal cellulitis. Eyelid abscesses require urgent surgical drainage, ideally by an ophthalmologist.

Dacryocystitis is not really an eyelid lump, but is discussed here because it presents as a mass close to the lower lid. The patient develops a tense, red, often painful swelling just inferior to the medial end of the lower eyelid (Figure 8.10). Dacryocystitis is due to infection of an obstructed lacrimal sac. Urgent ophthalmic referral is required.

Benign lid tumors include squamous papillomas (small, warty-looking lumps that are sometimes pedunculated) and compound nevi.

Malignant lid tumors include basal cell carcinoma (BCC), squamous cell carcinoma (SCC) and malignant melanoma. BCC and SCC of the eyelids can be life-threatening if they invade the orbit and reach the cavernous sinus; the risk of this happening is greatest if the lesion is in the medial eyelid. Melanoma is even more dangerous because it often metastasizes.

Figure 8.10 Dacryocystitis with pus discharge.

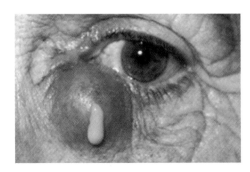

BCC presents as a pearly, telangiectatic nodule (Figure 8.11a), or less commonly as diffuse infiltration of the eyelid without a localized lesion.

SCC usually appears as a scaly lesion, sometimes with central ulceration.

Melanoma is usually a dark, flat or raised lid lesion, often with irregular margins (Figure 8.11b).

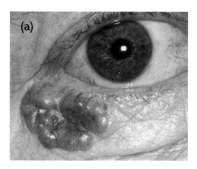 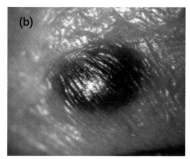

Figure 8.11 Malignant lid tumors: (a) basal cell carcinoma of the lower eyelid skin, presenting as a pearly, nodular growth; (b) melanoma of the eyelid skin.

Key points – eyelid disease

- Refer urgently, ideally to be seen by an ophthalmologist the same day, patients with one or more of:
  - acute unilateral or bilateral eyelid swelling with red eye and proptosis (possible orbital cellulitis)
  - any of the other signs of orbital cellulitis (see page 72)
  - preseptal cellulitis in a child, or in an adult if it does not settle with the use of oral antibiotics
  - acute onset of unilateral or bilateral ptosis with double vision, unequal pupils, body muscle weakness or problems with breathing or swallowing (possible myasthenia gravis or partial third nerve palsy from aneurysm or tumor)
  - herpes zoster ophthalmicus (shingles around the eye)
  - new-onset seventh nerve palsy of any cause.
- Refer semi-urgently any patient with suspected eyelid skin cancer, or entropion with eyelashes abrading the cornea.

In some ways, children's eye problems may have greater consequences than eye problems in adults, because some conditions, if neglected, may cause amblyopia ('lazy eye') which can reduce the vision in one or both eyes for the whole of the patient's life. In addition, life-threatening problems such as eye or brain tumors can, rarely, present with a squint ('turned eye'), poor red reflex or poor vision in an infant or child.

Referral

Urgent referral if your patient is:

- a neonate with red eyes and eye watering or discharge (possible ophthalmia neonatorum)
- a neonate/child with an abnormal red reflex (dull, absent or white)
- an infant/child with photophobia (without other signs of meningitis), corneal enlargement ('big eye/s') or cloudy cornea (possible congenital glaucoma)
- a child with red eye with pain, photophobia or blurred vision
- an older child with double vision (young children with idiopathic squints rarely have double vision, but in older children double vision has the same potentially serious causes as in adults)
- a child of any age with swollen optic disc/s on ophthalmoscopy

Semi-urgent referral for any child with:

- squint or nystagmus not yet assessed by an ophthalmologist
- visual field loss, or relative afferent pupillary defect (RAPD)
- suspected poor vision, or decreased visual acuity in one or both eyes that cannot be completely corrected with glasses
- red eye/s with normal vision and no pain or photophobia, which persists for longer than 2 weeks
- pale optic disc/s on ophthalmoscopy

Prompt referral to an ophthalmologist when indicated is essential if the potentially serious consequences of children's eye problems are to be avoided.

Routine referral is appropriate for:
- an infant with persisting eye watering or a slight sticky discharge from one or both eyes, with no eye redness, photophobia or corneal clouding or enlargement (likely to be congenital nasolacrimal duct obstruction)
- a child with a head tilt or turn (possible congenital fourth nerve palsy).

Eye discharge or watering
Most infants and children with 'watery' eyes have harmless congenital nasolacrimal duct obstruction; however, be careful not to miss the rare sight-threatening condition of congenital glaucoma, and the sight- and life-threatening disease ophthalmia neonatorum.

Ophthalmia neonatorum. In contrast with viral or bacterial conjunctivitis in children or adults, in whom the disease is annoying but rarely dangerous, conjunctivitis within the first few weeks of life (ophthalmia neonatorum) may be the first sign of a sight- or life-threatening systemic infection due to a sexually transmitted disease that the infant acquired during delivery.

Causative organisms include gonorrhea, chlamydia and herpes simplex virus (HSV) type II, which can also cause meningitis, encephalitis and other systemic infections. For this reason, neonates suspected of having ophthalmia neonatorum should be managed as an emergency by both a neonatologist and an ophthalmologist. Conjunctivitis alone (without systemic infection) can also be due to common, less virulent bacteria.

Congenital glaucoma is a rare but serious eye condition in which the child is born with persistent high pressure in one or both eyes. Congenital glaucoma does not cause red eyes, but does result in corneal and eye enlargement. Corneal clouding may develop, and the child may have constant watering of the eye/s and photophobia (aversion to bright lights). Prompt surgical treatment can save the child's sight.

Congenital nasolacrimal duct obstruction is very common. It presents as persistent watering or sticky discharge from one or both eyes, without eye redness, photophobia, or corneal enlargement or clouding. This often corrects itself within the first year to 18 months of life. Nasolacrimal duct probing under general anesthetic by an ophthalmologist can be performed after this time if the problem has not spontaneously resolved.

Conjunctivitis. Children of all ages may develop the usual types of conjunctivitis (viral, allergic and bacterial; see Chapter 2 – red eye).

Suspected poor vision

Young children are unable to complain of poor vision themselves, but parents may notice that their child is not looking at them or reacting to their facial expressions, or is having problems navigating and bumps into furniture. Poor vision in one or both eyes may also present with a noticeable squint or nystagmus (see overleaf). Assessing children's vision before they can talk may be difficult, but you can present them with various toys of different sizes and note their reaction, and observe how well they visually fix and follow the targets, as well as observing their general visual behavior.

A critical difference between childhood and adult vision is that children less than 9 years old with poor vision in one or both eyes from any cause, or one eye constantly turned from squint, will not develop normal connections between the affected eye/s and the developing visual cortex. This poor connection will result in permanent poor vision from amblyopia, even if the original eye problem is later corrected.

If, however, the cause of poor vision (e.g. congenital cataract) is treated urgently, permanent blindness from amblyopia may be prevented. In the case of squint, amblyopia may often be partially or fully corrected by patching the 'good' eye under close ophthalmic supervision. For these reasons, the ophthalmic assessment of children with poor vision is a matter of some urgency.

Abnormal red reflex or 'white pupil'

The normal red reflex seen with a direct ophthalmoscope in a dark room is a diffuse orange or red glow from both pupils.

A red reflex test is an essential part of every neonate's first medical examination after birth.

A red reflex test should be performed on any child with a squint, apparently poor vision or any other eye problem. If the red reflex on one or both sides is abnormal (Figure 9.1), a serious intraocular abnormality such as congenital cataract (dull or absent red reflex) or retinoblastoma (white reflex) is likely. Alternatively, you or the parents may notice that one or both pupils looks white or gray, rather than black.

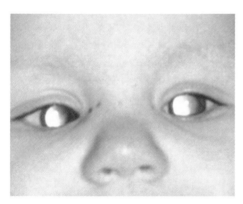

Figure 9.1 Bilateral abnormal (white) reflex in a child with bilateral retinoblastomas. Reproduced from Pane A, Simcock P. *Practical Ophthalmology: A Survival Guide for Doctors and Optometrists* with permission from Elsevier. Copyright © 2005.

Squint ('turned eye', strabismus)

Squint is never 'normal', and the vast majority of children with squint do not 'grow out' of it. Any child with a squint should be promptly referred to an ophthalmologist to determine its underlying cause.

Poor vision itself (including from a serious cause such as malignant retinoblastoma in one or both eyes, or congenital cataracts) can cause squint. Conversely, squint can cause poor vision, because an eye that is constantly turned will develop amblyopia. Children with squints usually do not (if they are old enough to talk) complain of double vision, because their brain 'switches off' the image from the deviated eye.

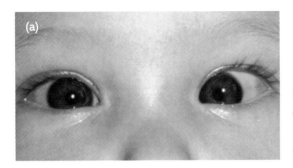

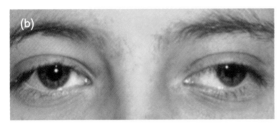

Figure 9.2 Common childhood squints: (a) idiopathic congenital esotropia; (b) idiopathic intermittent exotropia.

Children can develop squint from all the same causes as in adults, including third, fourth or sixth nerve palsies from brain tumor, inflammation or infection. However, by far the most common types of squint noticed within the first few years of life are the idiopathic childhood squints (Figure 9.2): infantile esotropia, accommodative esotropia and intermittent exotropia. These squints occur for an unknown reason in otherwise healthy children, and often can be partially or fully corrected with squint surgery, after refractive error has been treated with glasses and any amblyopia has been corrected with patching.

Nystagmus (continually moving eyes)

Children who are born bilaterally blind, or who develop blindness within the first few months of life (e.g. from congenital cataract or anterior visual pathway tumor), often develop constant movement of both eyes. Other children born with normal eyes and normal visual pathways develop nystagmus because of an inherited eye motor control problem. Nystagmus in children can also occur for all the same reasons as in adults, including brain tumors or middle-ear disease.

Optic disc abnormalities

Abnormal optic discs in children always require ophthalmic assessment. Swollen discs may represent papilledema due to a brain tumor or hydrocephalus. Pale discs may be associated with other congenital brain abnormalities or a tumor of the anterior visual pathway.

Key points – children's eye problems

- Refer urgently, ideally to be seen the same day, if your patient is:
  - a neonate with red eyes and eye watering or discharge (possible ophthalmia neonatorum)
  - a neonate or child with an abnormal red reflex (possible retinoblastoma or congenital cataract)
  - an infant or child with photophobia, corneal enlargement or cloudy cornea (possible congenital glaucoma)
  - a child with red eye with pain, photophobia or blurred vision (possible corneal ulcer, iritis or endophthalmitis)
  - an older child with double vision (causes include brain tumor or aneurysm)
  - a child of any age with swollen optic disc/s on ophthalmoscopy (possible brain tumor or hydrocephalus).
- Refer semi-urgently any child with:
  - squint ('turned eye', strabismus) or nystagmus (constantly moving eyes) not yet assessed by an ophthalmologist
  - visual field loss, or a relative afferent pupillary defect on the swinging light test (potentially serious optic nerve or brain disease)
  - suspected poor vision, or decreased visual acuity in one or both eyes, which cannot be completely corrected with glasses
  - red eye/s with normal vision and no pain or photophobia, which persists for longer than 2 weeks
  - pale optic disc/s on ophthalmoscopy.

Minor eye trauma is common and rarely serious – examples include corneal foreign body, corneal abrasion and periorbital bruising ('black eye'). However, all practitioners should also be able to recognize the warning symptoms and signs of serious eye trauma, including penetrating eye injury, intraocular foreign body and ruptured globe.

Referral

Immediate urgent referral of patients with serious eye trauma can save sight in the injured eye/s.

Urgent referral if your patient with eye trauma has:

- been hit in the eye by a high-speed metal fragment; even if you find a corneal foreign body or find no abnormality on examination, the patient needs an X-ray to exclude the presence of an intraocular foreign body
- unexplained eye pain, blurred vision, photophobia, flashes, floaters, field loss or double vision
- an unexplained decrease in visual acuity (VA), field defect to confrontation, relative afferent pupillary defect, unexplained red eye, visible abnormality of the cornea, abnormal pupil shape or size, absent red reflex or swollen optic disc/s
- blood in the anterior chamber (hyphema)
- eyelids that are swollen shut, so that you cannot test VA (an ultrasound or computed tomography [CT] scan may be needed to confirm that the eyeball is intact)
- chemical or thermal burn to the eyes
- a suspected infectious ulcer that has developed around a corneal foreign body
- a non-infected corneal abrasion that has not healed within 3 days

You can treat the following conditions yourself, although you will need to refer them if the problem persists or worsens:

- corneal foreign body (if you are confident treating this)
- foreign body under the upper lid
- corneal abrasion with no sign of penetrating eye injury or infection
- subconjunctival hemorrhage with no other eye abnormalities
- 'black eye' with no other eye symptoms, normal VA and an examination that is normal apart from eyelid bruising.

Serious eye injuries

A patient suspected of having any of these injuries requires urgent referral.

Penetrating eye injury. Direct trauma with a sharp object may lacerate the cornea or sclera (Figure 10.1). Ocular structures are often damaged at the time, but there is also a high risk of intraocular infection that can cause blindness and loss of the eye within days. Injuries range from the eye being struck with the sharp tip of a palm frond while gardening, which may result in an eye with normal vision that has a barely visible corneal laceration, to a patient whose eye has been severely lacerated with broken glass.

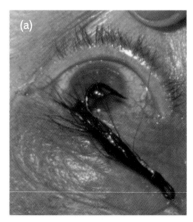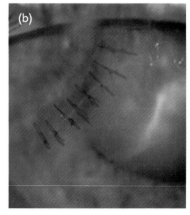

Figure 10.1 (a) Penetrating eye injury. (b) Corneal sutures following surgical repair of a perforation from a fly fishing hook.

Warning symptoms and signs (which are not always present) to watch out for include:

- complaints of pain, blurred vision, floaters or field loss after a suspicious-sounding injury
- a distorted pupil (teardrop shape with the point due to iris prolapse at the site of penetration)
- hyphema (blood in the anterior chamber).

Telephone an ophthalmologist immediately if you suspect your patient has a penetrating eye injury.

> It is important to suspect a penetrating injury in any patient with a suggestive history. Even if the eye looks normal on examination, you must refer the patient urgently because of the risk of intraocular infection.

Intraocular foreign body is most commonly caused by a small piece of high-speed metal striking the eye, often in metalworkers whilst hammering. Again, you need to maintain a high index of suspicion even if the eye looks normal to you and even if you find a corneal foreign body, as a second piece of metal could be inside the eye. An urgent slit-lamp examination and X-ray of the orbit should be carried out in any patient who says they have been hit in the eye with a high-speed fragment.

If an intraocular foreign body is not detected and surgically removed early, loss of the eye through infection can occur. Hammering metal is the classic cause of an intraocular foreign body; fragments from grinding metal more commonly result in superficial foreign bodies.

Ruptured globe. Severe blunt trauma may split the sclera open, but because the overlying conjunctiva may remain intact this type of injury is often not directly visible on examination. The patient usually complains of severe pain, blurred vision and often floaters (due to vitreous hemorrhage) or field loss (due to retinal detachment). Intraocular pressure is often low.

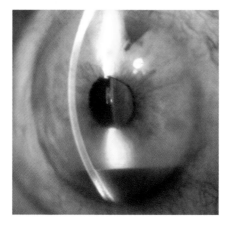

Figure 10.2 Hyphema – blood in the anterior chamber.

Hyphema is blood in the anterior chamber (between the cornea and the iris) (Figure 10.2). Hyphema may be seen after blunt trauma that has caused no other damage to the eye, or it may be a sign of penetrating eye injury, intraocular foreign body or ruptured globe. The major risk to sight after isolated hyphema (with no other eye damage) is high intraocular pressure, which can cause damage to the optic nerve head or retinal vascular occlusion. Permanent corneal blood staining can also occur.

Orbital fracture. The most common fracture is an orbital floor 'blowout' fracture, which is often seen on X-ray or CT scan as a fluid level in the maxillary sinus, or as soft tissue protruding into the sinus from the orbital floor (Figure 10.3). Air in the orbit may also be seen. This injury should be suspected in any patient with blunt facial trauma who admits to double vision or a numb cheek or numb upper teeth on the side of the injury.

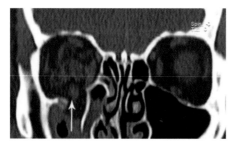

Figure 10.3 Computed tomography scan of an orbital floor blowout fracture, with tissue prolapse into the maxillary antrum (arrowed).

Chemical burn. Strong alkalis in particular may cause devastating damage to the eye, often resulting in blindness or loss of the eye. However, mild chemical burns are more common (e.g. from shampoo, washing detergent and so on), and cause mild discomfort but are not dangerous.

It is essential that, in all cases of suspected chemical burn, the patient irrigates the affected eye/s under running water or saline for 30 minutes as a matter of urgency. Irrigate the eye/s yourself if the patient has not adequately done so already before arriving at your practice.

> Irrigation must be performed immediately – do not delay by examining the eye first, or testing the pH with paper test strips.

If the patient is in severe discomfort, several drops of topical anesthetic will allow more comfortable irrigation.

All patients with possible eye chemical burn who initially had significant pain, photophobia or blurred vision require urgent ophthalmic referral for slit-lamp examination and treatment (even if their eyes look normal on examination).

Thermal burn. Flame burns to the face may seriously damage the eyes; in addition, associated respiratory burns may cause life-threatening complications later. For this reason, any patient with flame burns to the face requires urgent ambulance transfer to a general emergency department for systemic workup; an ophthalmologist will be consulted once life-threatening injuries have been excluded.

Eyelid laceration. Because of the functional and cosmetic importance of the eyelids, these injuries should ideally be repaired by an ophthalmologist or plastic surgeon within 24 hours. Remember also to perform a careful eye examination, as there may also be a penetrating eye injury. Consult an ophthalmologist for medial upper or lower lid lacerations, because the lacrimal drainage apparatus in the medial eyelid margin may have been lacerated and require special repair.

Minor eye injuries

These can still develop into major problems if they are not treated appropriately. The patient should be referred immediately if the problem persists or worsens.

Corneal foreign body (Figure 10.4) is common and often seen in workers who have been grinding metal. The patient complains of foreign body sensation and/or mild pain and photophobia. If the pain and photophobia are severe, you should suspect a superimposed infectious corneal ulcer and refer the patient immediately.

Some corneal foreign bodies are loose and can be carefully wiped off with a sterile cotton swab (cotton bud) after the eye has been numbed with local anesthetic drops. If the foreign body is more adherent, it requires removal with a fine sterile needle. Only do this if you have previously been shown what to do, as it is possible to perforate the cornea if you are not careful. If the foreign body cannot be completely removed, refer the patient to an ophthalmologist within 24 hours ('trying again' yourself the next day usually does not help) – you can apply antibiotic ointment and a pressure patch in the meantime for comfort.

If you have been able to fully remove the foreign body, apply antibiotic ointment and a pressure patch (double eye pad) and review the patient the next day. The small corneal abrasion caused by removal of a foreign body should be reviewed daily with blue light and fluorescein drops, and should be seen to heal completely within 3 days. If it does not heal within this time or if the patient develops increasing pain or photophobia, refer urgently as infection could be present.

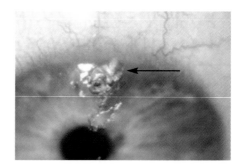

Figure 10.4 Corneal foreign body (arrowed).

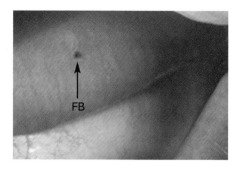

Figure 10.5 Foreign body under the upper lid. FB, subtarsal foreign body.

Foreign body under the upper lid can cause foreign body sensation and irritation, and occasionally corneal ulcer by abrading the underlying cornea. The patient may or may not remember anything going into the eye, and the foreign body will not be discovered unless the upper lid is everted (Figure 10.5). For this reason, remember to evert the upper lid in all patients who present with unexplained foreign body sensation (see Chapter 1 – eye examination). The foreign body is usually easily wiped away with a cotton swab (cotton bud).

Corneal abrasion is focal loss of the thin surface layer (epithelium) of the cornea, with no laceration of the main substance of the cornea. Abrasions are frequently caused by scratches or minor blunt trauma to the eye, and often cause intense pain and foreign body sensation. The abrasion may be invisible unless a blue light and fluorescein is used (Figure 10.6); the eye should be otherwise normal and have no signs of corneal laceration or penetrating eye injury. If you have any doubt, refer urgently for a slit-lamp examination.

Figure 10.6 Corneal abrasion that stains with fluorescein dye when examined with a blue light.

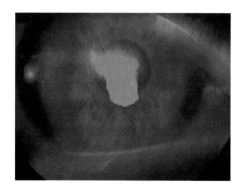

If you are confident that an isolated corneal abrasion is present, with no signs of infection (the corneal substance underneath the abrasion remains completely clear, rather than cloudy or white as occurs in infectious ulcers), apply antibiotic ointment and a pressure patch. You will need to review and repatch the eye daily until it has healed. If the abrasion does not heal completely within 3 days, refer urgently.

Subconjunctival hemorrhage looks startling, but is not serious unless there are other underlying injuries (such as a penetrating eye injury). The layer of bright red blood between the clear conjunctiva and white sclera resolves over a few weeks (see Figure 2.10, page 29). No treatment is needed if no other injuries are present.

'Black eye' is bruising of the eyelids due to blunt trauma. It is not serious and will resolve spontaneously; however, it is possible to miss an underlying serious eye injury, such as hyphema or ruptured globe, because of difficulty examining the eye (the eyelids may be so swollen that they prevent eye examination, or the patient may be drunk or uncooperative).

It is essential that you measure VA in every patient with a 'black eye', and carry out as full an eye examination as is possible. Even if the eyelids are severely swollen it is usually possible to prise them apart with cotton swabs (cotton buds) to obtain a VA measurement. If the initial examination reveals no serious eye injury, review the patient for re-examination in a few days. On repeat visits, check that the patient is not experiencing double vision (this may only be noticed as lid swelling recedes).

If you see the patient immediately after the injury, advise them to apply ice packs to the swollen eyelids and to sleep with their head elevated, which will reduce the swelling more quickly. Tell them to avoid taking aspirin for analgesia as this may increase bruising.

Key points – eye trauma

- Refer urgently, to be seen by an ophthalmologist the same day, if your patient with eye trauma has:
  - been hit in the eye by a high-speed metal fragment; even if you find a corneal foreign body or find no abnormality on examination, the patient needs an X-ray to exclude the presence of an intraocular foreign body
  - unexplained eye pain, blurred vision, photophobia, flashes, floaters, field loss or double vision
  - an unexplained decrease in visual acuity (VA), field defect to confrontation, relative afferent pupillary defect, unexplained red eye, visible abnormality of the cornea, abnormal pupil shape or size, absent red reflex or swollen optic disc/s
  - blood in the anterior chamber (hyphema)
  - eyelids that are swollen shut, so that you cannot test VA (an ultrasound or computed tomography scan may be needed to confirm that the eyeball is intact)
  - chemical or thermal burn to the eyes
  - a suspected infectious ulcer that has developed around a corneal foreign body
  - a non-infectious corneal abrasion that has not healed within 3 days.

Useful resources

Further reading
Kanski JJ. *Clinical Ophthalmology*, 5th edn. Oxford: Butterworth Heinemann, 2003.

Pane A, Simcock P. *Practical Ophthalmology: A Survival Guide for Doctors and Optometrists*. Edinburgh: Churchill Livingstone, 2005.

Patient support groups
International Glaucoma Association
(Registered charity offering advice and support to glaucoma sufferers)
Woodcote House
15 Highpoint Business Village
Henwood, Ashford
Kent TN24 8DH
Sightline: 0870 609 1870
Tel: +44 (0)1233 648170
Fax: +44 (0)1233 648179
info@iga.org.uk
www.iga.org.uk

Macular Disease Society (UK)
(Self-help society providing information and practical support for people with macular disease)
PO Box 1870
Andover, Hampshire SP10 9AD
Helpline: 0845 241 2041
Tel: +44 (0)1264 350551
Fax: +44 (0)1264 350558
info@maculardisease.org
www.maculardisease.org

Prevent Blindness America
(Voluntary eye health and safety organization)
211 West Wacker Drive
Suite 1700
Chicago, IL 60606
Helpline: 1 800 331 2020
(8.30 AM–5 PM CST, Mon–Fri)
info@preventblindness.org
www.preventblindness.org

Royal National Institute of the Blind (UK)
105 Judd Street
London WC1H 9NE
Helpline: 0845 766 9999
(9 AM–5 PM, Mon–Fri)
Tel: +44 (0)20 7388 1266
Fax: +44 (0)20 7388 2034
helpline@rnib.org.uk
www.rnib.org.uk

Royal Society for the Blind
(South Australia)
254 Angas Street
Adelaide SA 5000
Tel: +61 (0)8 8223 6222
Fax: +61 (0)8 8223 7836
www.rsb.org.au

Vision Australia
(National blindness agency)
4 Mitchell Street
Enfield NSW 2136
Tel: 1300 847466
Fax: +61 (0)2 9747 5993
info@visionaustralia.org.au
www.visionaustralia.org.au

Professional organizations

American Academy of
Ophthalmology
PO Box 7424
San Francisco, CA 94120-7424
Tel: +1 415 561 8500
Fax: +1 415 561 8533
www.aao.org

International Council of
Ophthalmology (USA)
c/o Bruce E Spivey MD
Secretary-General
945 Green Street
San Francisco, CA 94133
Fax: +1 415 409 403
info@icoph.org
www.icoph.org

Royal Australian and New Zealand
College of Ophthalmologists
94–98 Chalmers Street
Surrey Hills, NSW 2010
Australia
Tel: +61 (0)2 9690 1001
Fax: +61 (0)2 9690 1321
ranzco@ranzco.edu
www.ranzco.edu

Royal College of
Ophthalmologists (UK)
17 Cornwall Terrace
London NW1 4QW
Tel: +44 (0)20 7935 0702
Fax: +44 (0)20 7935 9838
www.rcophth.ac.uk

Index